O A I D L
OXFORD AMERICAN INFECTIOUS DISEASE LIBRARY

The New Hepatitis C

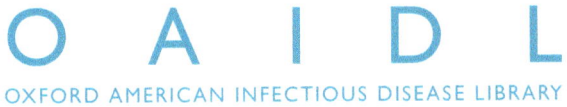

OXFORD AMERICAN INFECTIOUS DISEASE LIBRARY

The New Hepatitis C

Effective Clinical Management in the Age of All-Oral Therapy

Second Edition

Edited by

Nancy Reau

Donald M. Jensen

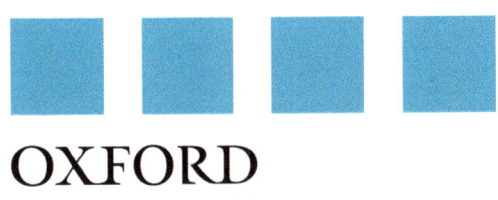

OXFORD
UNIVERSITY PRESS

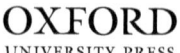

Oxford University Press is a department of the University of Oxford. It furthers
the University's objective of excellence in research, scholarship, and education
by publishing worldwide. Oxford is a registered trade mark of Oxford University
Press in the UK and certain other countries.

Published in the United States of America by Oxford University Press
198 Madison Avenue, New York, NY 10016, United States of America.

© Oxford University Press 2018

First Edition published in 2013
Second Edition published in 2018

All rights reserved. No part of this publication may be reproduced, stored in
a retrieval system, or transmitted, in any form or by any means, without the
prior permission in writing of Oxford University Press, or as expressly permitted
by law, by license, or under terms agreed with the appropriate reproduction
rights organization. Inquiries concerning reproduction outside the scope of the
above should be sent to the Rights Department, Oxford University Press, at the
address above.

You must not circulate this work in any other form
and you must impose this same condition on any acquirer.

Library of Congress Cataloging-in-Publication Data
Names: Reau, Nancy, editor. | Jensen, Donald, editor.
Title: The new Hepatitis C : effective clinical management in the age of all-oral therapy /
edited by Nancy Reau, Donald Jensen.
Other titles: Hepatitis C | Oxford American infectious disease library.
Description: Second edition. | Oxford ; New York : Oxford University Press, [2018] |
Series: Oxford American infectious disease library | Preceded by Hepatitis C /
[edited by] Donald Jensen, Nancy Reau. 2013. |
Includes bibliographical references and index.
Identifiers: LCCN 2017038174 | ISBN 9780190238285 (pbk)
Subjects: | MESH: Hepatitis C | Hepatitis C—drug therapy |
Antiviral Agents—therapeutic use
Classification: LCC RC848.H425 | NLM WC 536 | DDC 616.3/623—dc23
LC record available at https://lccn.loc.gov/2017038174

This material is not intended to be, and should not be considered, a substitute for medical
or other professional advice. Treatment for the conditions described in this material is highly
dependent on the individual circumstances. And, while this material is designed to offer
accurate information with respect to the subject matter covered and to be current as of the
time it was written, research and knowledge about medical and health issues is constantly
evolving and dose schedules for medications are being revised continually, with new side
effects recognized and accounted for regularly. Readers must therefore always check the
product information and clinical procedures with the most up- to- date published product
information and data sheets provided by the manufacturers and the most recent codes
of conduct and safety regulation. The publisher and the authors make no representations
or warranties to readers, express or implied, as to the accuracy or completeness of
this material. Without limiting the foregoing, the publisher and the authors make no
representations or warranties as to the accuracy or efficacy of the drug dosages mentioned
in the material. The authors and the publisher do not accept, and expressly disclaim, any
responsibility for any liability, loss, or risk that may be claimed or incurred as a consequence
of the use and/ or application of any of the contents of this material

Disclosures

Andres F. Carrion has served as a scientific advisor to Gilead and has received speakers' honoraria from Merck and Bristol Myers-Squibb. Stanley Martin Cohen is on speakers bureaus and advisory boards for Gilead and Abbvie. Steven L. Flamm has served as a research consultant for Gilead, Merck, and Abbvie. Josh Levitsky has served as a speaker for Gilead science. Paul Martin has served as an investigator for Gilead, Merck, and Abbvie and as a consultant for Gilead and Abbvie. He is on Bristol-Myers Squibb's Data Safety Monitoring Board. Nancy Reau has served as a scientific advisor to Abbott, Abbvie, Gilead, and Merck, and her institution has received funding from Abbott, Abbvie, and Gilead. Rohit Satoskar is on the speaker bureau for Gilead, serves as a consultant for Gilead, and has received research grants from Gilead and Merck. Helen S. Te has received research support from Abbvie. All other contributors have nothing to disclose.

Preface

Rapid and profound changes are taking place in the field of hepatitis C therapeutics. Not only is all-oral interferon-free therapy a possibility, it has become the standard of care for all patients across genotype, cirrhosis status, and comorbid conditions in most countries. Cure rates of higher than 95% are now commonplace. And even those who fail first attempts at therapy have all-oral options with high expectations for viral eradication.

More than ever, these rapid therapeutic changes compel us to review the broader scope of hepatitis C, including its epidemiology, diagnostics, natural history, and clinical features. It is only through recognition of those at risk that screening efforts can lead to successful control of hepatitis C. For the first time in history, elimination of the hepatitis C virus (HCV) is viewed as an achievable goal.

Given the accelerated advance in hepatitis C knowledge, a review of these features can help assist in this common target. Our goal in the preparation of this handbook is to provide the fundamentals of our knowledge of hepatitis C to allow readers to quickly survey the field, yet with the confidence that the information is current and accurate.

The first five chapters provide the framework for the more clinical chapters to come. Chapter 1 describes in clear and understandable terms the basic biology of HCV. It is this information that has led to the development of direct-acting antiviral agents and is thus essential reading. Chapter 2 discusses the epidemiology of hepatitis C, including the geographic prevalence of the various HCV genotypes—an important consideration given globalization and international travel. Chapter 3 covers the natural history of HCV, including current information regarding risk factors for transmission. Diagnostic testing for HCV is presented in Chapter 4, which includes a concise overview of nucleic acid testing limitations and use. Chapter 5, details the histopathologic features of acute and chronic HCV infection and the importance of the grading scale used to define inflammatory and fibrosis components, with excellent graphics to help those less familiar with pathology. These first five chapters represent the key background information on which most clinical decision-making is based.

The relatively uncommon but important issue of acute hepatitis C is discussed in Chapter 6, including the serologic diagnosis. Chronic hepatitis C is reviewed in Chapter 7, providing an overview and recapitulation of its natural history. The importance and evaluation of the extrahepatic manifestations of chronic hepatitis C are elaborated in Chapter 8.

Chapters 9 and 10 cover therapy for both treatment-naïve and treatment-experienced individuals. This is followed by a thorough review of the issues facing special populations in Chapter 11, with Chapter 12 covering aspects pertinent to liver transplantation.

Chapter 13 emphasizes that the care of the patient with HCV does not end with viral eradication. Finally, Chapter 14 provides a useful review of the lexicon of the numerous clinical trials in HCV.

We hope that readers will find this book both informative and clinically useful. We have attempted to keep verbiage to a minimum while presenting key points in easily referenced tables. In a rapidly moving field, this book offers the reader a valuable pocket resource for years to come.

Contents

Contributors *xi*

1. Basic Virology of Hepatitis C — 1
   Glenn Randall
2. Epidemiology of Hepatitis C — 7
   Adam E. Mikolajczyk and Helen S. Te
3. Natural History of Hepatitis C — 17
   Cassandra Fritz and Andrew Aronsohn
4. Diagnostic Testing for Hepatitis C — 33
   Natasha von Roenn
5. Pathology of Viral Hepatitis C — 43
   Shriram Jakate
6. Acute Hepatitis C — 57
   Christin N. Price and Arthur Y. Kim
7. Chronic Hepatitis C — 65
   Rohit Satoskar and Tenzin Choden
8. Extrahepatic Manifestations of Hepatitis C — 75
   Suzanne Robertazzi and Anjana A. Pillai
9. Treatment of Hepatitis C Genotypes 1, 4, 5, 6 — 83
   Ramakrishna Behara and Steven L. Flamm
10. Treatment of Hepatitis C Genotypes 2 and 3 — 91
    Deepak Venkat and Stanley Martin Cohen
11. Treatment of Hepatitis C in Special Populations — 111
    Andres F. Carrion and Paul Martin
12. Hepatitis C in Liver Transplantation — 131
    Justin R. Boike and Josh Levitsky
13. Management of Hepatitis C After a Cure — 149
    Daniel Berger and Sheila Eswaran

14. Lexicon of Trials 155
   Deeksha Seth, Sujit V. Janardhan, and Archita P. Desai

   Index *181*

Contributors

Andrew Aronsohn, MD
Associate Professor of Medicine
University of Chicago Center for
Liver Diseases
University of Chicago Medicine

Ramakrishna Behara, DO
Gastroenterologist
Renaissance Gastroenterology

Daniel Berger, MD
Fellow, Gastroenterology and
Hepatology
Rush University Medical Center

Justin R. Boike, MD, MPH
Fellow, Gastroenterology and
Hepatology
Northwestern University

Andres F. Carrion, MD
Director of Hepatology
Assistant Professor of Medicine
Texas Tech University Health
Sciences Center

Tenzin Choden, MD
Resident Physician, Internal Medicine
MedStar Georgetown University
Hospital

Stanley Martin Cohen, MD, FAASLD, FACG
Professor of Medicine
Medical Director of Hepatology
University Hospitals/Cleveland
Medical Center

Archita P. Desai, MD
Assistant Professor of Medicine
Thomas D. Boyer Liver Institute
University of Arizona

Sheila Eswaran, MD, MS
Assistant Professor of Internal
Medicine Section
of Hepatology
Rush University Medical Center

Steven L. Flamm, MD
Professor of Medicine
and Surgery
Feinberg School of Medicine
Northwestern University

Cassandra Fritz, MD
Resident Physician
Barnes Jewish Hospital

Shriram Jakate, MD, FRCPath
Professor of Pathology
Gastroenterology
and Hepatology
Rush University Medical Center

Sujit V. Janardhan, MD, PhD
Assistant Professor of Medicine
Section of Hepatology
Rush University Medical Center

Arthur Y. Kim, MD
Associate Professor
of Medicine
Harvard Medical School
Director, Viral Hepatitis Clinic
Division of Infectious Diseases
Massachusetts General Hospital

Josh Levitsky, MD
Professor of Medicine
and Surgery
Feinberg School of Medicine
Northwestern University

Paul Martin, MD, FRCP, FRCPI
Chief, Gastroenterology and Hepatology
Professor of Medicine
Miller School of Medicine
University of Miami

Adam E. Mikolajczyk, MD
Transplant Hepatology Fellow
University of Chicago Medicine

Anjana A. Pillai, MD
Associate Professor of Medicine
Medical Director, Liver Tumor Clinic
University of Chicago Medicine

Christin N. Price, MD
Department of Internal Medicine
Brigham and Women's Hospital

Glenn Randall, PhD
Associate Professor of Microbiology
Biological Sciences Division
University of Chicago

Suzanne Robertazzi, CRNP
Transplant Institute
MedStar Georgetown University Hospital

Rohit Satoskar, MD
Associate Professor
Department of Medicine
Medical Director
of Transplantation
Transplant Institute
MedStar Georgetown University Hospital

Deeksha Seth, MBBS
Kasturba Medical College
Manipal University

Helen S. Te, MD
Professor of Medicine
Medical Director of Liver Transplanation
University of Chicago Medicine

Deepak Venkat, MD
Division of Gastroenterology
Henry Ford Health System

Natasha von Roenn, MD
Assistant Professor of Medicine
Division of Hepatology
Loyola University Medical Center

Chapter 1

Basic Virology of Hepatitis C

Glenn Randall

The Virus

Hepatitis C virus (HCV) is a major public health problem, with an estimated 71 million chronically infected people globally and 3 million in the United States.[1] It is one of multiple hepatitis viruses that are not genetically related to each other but share the property of causing disease of the liver. HCV is a blood-borne pathogen, requiring exchange of contaminated blood for efficient transmission. It was a major cause of non-A/non-B hepatitis, acquired primarily through tainted blood, until its discovery in 1989 enabled screening of the blood supply. Since the effective elimination of HCV from the blood supply, a major source on new infections is intravenous drug users sharing contaminated needles. This population is also at high risk for co-infection with hepatitis B virus and/or human immunodeficiency virus (HIV).

Patients with HCV can remain asymptomatic for long periods of time. Eventually, however, approximately 20% of patients will develop cirrhosis of the liver. Cirrhotic patients have a 2–4% annual rate of progression to end-stage liver disease or liver cancer. As such, HCV is a major cause of liver transplantation. There is no vaccine for HCV, and prior drug treatments for HCV, which targeted human proteins, had mixed success with serious associated side effects. Recently developed drugs that target viral proteins produce remarkable cure rates of greater than 95%.[2] The drugs are actually cocktails of different drugs that typically target multiple HCV proteins, including NS5A and NS5B, and sometimes NS3.

The virus structure, called a virion, is shown in Figure 1.1. Unlike humans, the genetic material of HCV is ribonucleic acid (RNA). The genome is one long RNA strand containing approximately 9,600 nucleotides.[3] The RNA is protected from the environment by a protein shell called a *capsid*. Surrounding the capsid is a lipid membrane called an *envelope*. The envelope is acquired from human membranes and contains the viral envelope proteins E1 and E2. The envelope proteins bind receptor proteins on human liver cells to initiate infection. The size of the HCV virions varies, but are approximately 60 nanometers in diameter. One reason that it has been historically difficult to develop antiviral drugs, as opposed to antibiotics that target bacteria, is that the viral envelope is covered in our own membrane and thus is not chemically distinct from our own cells. Bacterial cell walls are chemically different and can be targeted by drugs like penicillin.

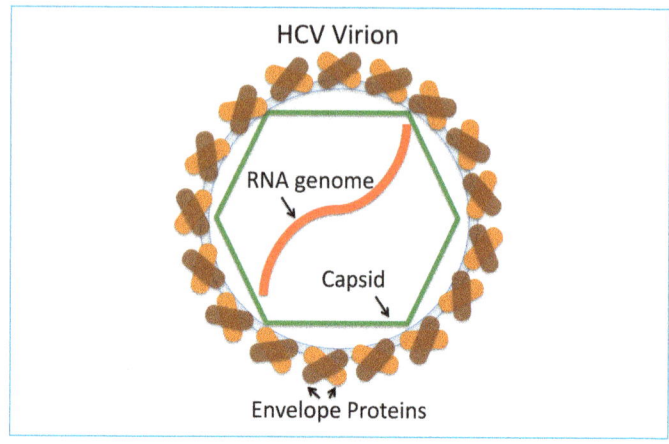

Figure 1.1 The HCV virion

Viruses are simple genetically and do not contain all of the information they need to replicate. Instead, they depend on human cells to perform some of the key functions in the viral life cycle. For instance, viruses are not capable of producing proteins since they do not contain ribosomes. Instead they use cellular ribosomes to make their proteins. This is another reason why antiviral drugs are difficult to develop, as opposed to antibiotics. Bacteria have their own protein synthesis machinery that is different from ours and that can be specifically targeted. Since viruses use many cellular functions, it is more difficult to selectively target them without harming the patient.

HCV Quasispecies and Genotypes

There is a great amount of variation in the RNA sequences of HCV genomes, shown in Figure 1.2. This is due in part to its mode of replication. DNA genomes are relatively static because the enzymes that synthesize DNA, called *DNA polymerases*, have proofreading activity. They can recognize mistakes in the DNA sequence and edit them. RNA genomes are less static because RNA polymerases lack proofreading activity. The HCV RNA polymerase makes a mistake once every 10,000 nucleotides, which coincidentally is about the size of its genome. Thus, each new viral genome contains approximately one different base from its parent virus. These mutations can either be detrimental by disrupting an essential viral function; neutral; or, in some cases, beneficial, as described later.

A chronically infected individual produces approximately 10^{12} HCV genomes every day, most of which vary slightly from each other due to these polymerase mistakes.[4] These variant viruses within the same infected person are called *quasispecies*. HCV quasispecies present a formidable challenge to treating infection. Although the virus variants are similar to each other, sometimes the small differences can have a major impact on a virus evading

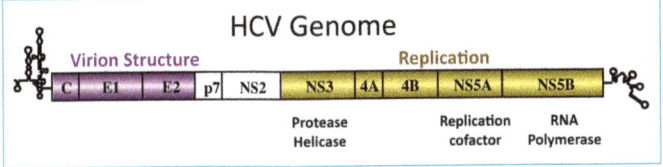

Figure 1.2 The HCV genome

the immune system or developing drug resistance. Our adaptive immune response to HCV produces antibodies that bind HCV virions to prevent infection and T-cell responses, which kill infected cells that are presenting parts of viral proteins on their surface. These immune responses typically target the most abundant virus variants and are effective at eliminating them. However, rare HCV variants that contain mutations in the parts of the proteins that are recognized by the immune system are not controlled by the immune system. These variants become dominant in the infected person until they, in turn, are subsequently targeted by immune cells. Then a new resistant HCV variant emerges. This evolutionary "arms race" between the virus and the immune system is a hallmark of chronic viral infections.

Quasispecies are also a problem with antiviral drug resistance. Minor HCV variants that are not sensitive to the drug can be selected, as just described. This is the reason that single drugs are no longer used to treat HIV or HCV. It is too easy for drug resistance to emerge. However, when drugs that target different viral proteins or functions are combined, then resistance is less likely to emerge. It is mathematically less likely for a virus to acquire all of the mutations to become resistant to multiple drugs.

As HCV has evolved in the population, the variations in genome sequences have become more dramatic. HCV has been classified into seven genotypes, which vary from each other by more than 30% at the nucleotide level.[4] Viruses within the same genotype are more similar in sequence to each other than they are to an HCV isolate from a different genotype. These genotypes are thought to largely reflect the geographical distribution of the virus. The genotype of the virus can also affect the response to therapy. Thus, the genotype of the virus has been an important criterion when evaluating which therapy a patient should receive.[5] In June 2016, the first drug that is effective against all HCV genotypes, Epclusa, was approved by the US Food and Drug Administration (FDA). It is a combination of NS5A and NS5B inhibitors.

HCV Replication and Drug Targets

HCV completes its life cycle in a liver cell, shown in Figure 1.3, in approximately 1 day.[3] It first infects liver cells by directly engaging a series of cellular proteins, called *receptors*, which are expressed on the outside surface of liver cells. The virion enters the liver cell following receptor binding and is delivered to enclosed compartments called *endosomes*. When the endosomes reach an acidic pH, the virion envelope fuses with the endosome and the virion uncoats, delivering its RNA genome into the cytoplasm of cells. The beginning of the viral genome contains an RNA structure that directly

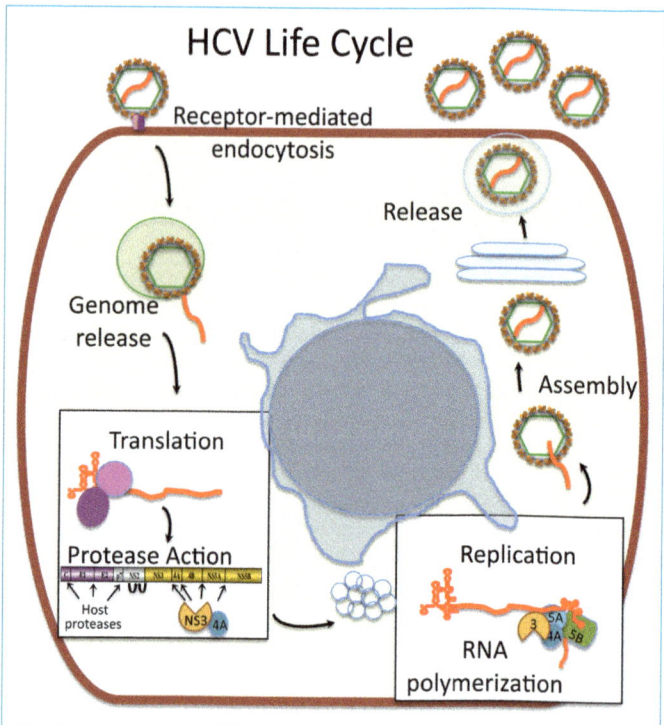

Figure 1.3 The HCV life cycle

binds human ribosomes, which initiates the translation of the HCV genome into one long protein. This long protein is then cut into at least 10 individual proteins by enzymes that are called *proteases*. The long HCV protein is cut by cellular and viral proteases. The viral NS3 protease is a target for some HCV drugs. These drugs typically bind NS3 near its active site and prevent its ability to cut the long HCV protein into individual proteins. Without protease cleavage, HCV is unable to replicate.

Once the individual proteins are produced, viral replication can initiate. The viral proteins NS3, NS4A, NS4B, NS5A, and NS5B are thought to form a replication complex. NS5B performs a critical function in replication: it is the RNA-dependent RNA polymerase. This means that it uses RNA as a template to synthesize new RNA. HCV replicates through a double-stranded RNA intermediate. The replication complex binds to the end of the HCV genome, and then NS5B synthesizes a complementary RNA strand called the *minus strand*. The minus strand can then in turn be used to serve as a template for the synthesis of HCV genomic RNAs. These genomic RNAs can either be translated to make more HCV proteins, or, alternatively, they are assembled into virions. These virions then leave the cell by the secretory pathway and are released from the cell to initiate infection of a new cell.

The activity of the NS5B polymerase is the second major target of new HCV drugs. There are different ways to inhibit replication. The first are called *nucleoside* or *nucleotide analogues*. These resemble RNA nucleotides that are incorporated into the newly synthesized viral RNA, but they lack chemical features that are required for linking new nucleotides to it. Thus, the elongating RNA is stopped, a process referred to as *chain termination*. One of the most effective HCV dugs, sofosbuvir, belongs to this drug class.[6] A second mechanism of polymerase inhibition is nucleoside-like drugs that compete with real nucleotides for binding to the polymerase. Finally, some drugs bind the polymerase outside of its active site and alter the structure of the polymerase so that it no longer functions.[7]

The final major drug target for treating HCV is NS5A. A screen of a chemical library for compounds that inhibit HCV replication identified NS5A inhibitors.[8] One such drug that works at very low concentrations is thought to target NS5A because mutations that produce resistance to the drug map to NS5A. NS5A has multiple roles in the viral life cycle, including establishing replication compartments, aiding the polymerase in replication, and assembling virions. NS5A inhibitors interfere with many of these processes, including the replication compartment formation and virion assembly. These drugs represent a critical component of anti-HCV drug cocktails, most frequently combined with NS5B polymerase inhibitors.

References

1. Global Hepatitis Report, 2017 (n.d.). Available: http://www.who.int/hepatitis/publications/global-hepatitis-report2017/en/.

2. Pawlotsky JM, Feld JJ, Zeuzem S, Hoofnagle JH. From non-A, non-B hepatitis to hepatitis C virus cure. *J Hepatol*. 2015;62:S87–S99.

3. Moradpour D, Penin F, Rice CM. Replication of hepatitis C virus. *Nat Rev Microbiol*. 2007;5:453–463.

4. Smith DB, Bukh J, Kuiken C, et al. Expanded classification of hepatitis C virus into 7 genotypes and 67 subtypes: updated criteria and genotype assignment web resource. *Hepatology*. 2013;59:318–327. doi:10.1002/hep.26744

5. Jacobson IM. The HCV treatment revolution continues: resistance considerations, pangenotypic efficacy, and advances in challenging populations. *Gastroenterol Hepatol (N Y)*. 2016;12:1–11.

6. Lawitz E, Jacobson IM, Nelson DR, et al. Development of sofosbuvir for the treatment of hepatitis C virus infection. *Ann N Y Acad Sci*. 2015;1358:56–67.

7. De Francesco R, Migliaccio G. Challenges and successes in developing new therapies for hepatitis C. *Nature*. 2005;436:953–960.

8. Gao M, Nettles RE, Belema M, et al. Chemical genetics strategy identifies an HCV NS5A inhibitor with a potent clinical effect. *Nature*. 2010;465:96–100.

Chapter 2

Epidemiology of Hepatitis C

Adam E. Mikolajczyk and Helen S. Te

Introduction

Hepatitis C virus (HCV) is an RNA virus known to infect humans and chimpanzees, causing a similar disease in these two species. It is the most common cause of transfusion-related hepatitis and is one of the leading causes of end-stage liver disease requiring liver transplantation in the United States. It is transmitted most efficiently by parenteral means, particularly with large or repeated exposure to infected blood products or transplantation of infected tissue or organ grafts, and intravenous drug use (IVDU). Less frequently, it can be transmitted by mucosal exposures to blood or serum-derived fluids through perinatal or sexual means.[1]

The relative mutability of its genome has been blamed for its high propensity to cause chronic infection. About 80% of new infections progress to chronic infection, with cirrhosis developing in about 20% of infected individuals after 20–30 years, resulting in increased risk for liver failure, portal hypertension–related complications, and hepatocellular carcinoma (HCC). The high mutability of the HCV genome and limited knowledge in the protective immune response following infection has hindered progress in vaccine development. For this reason, no vaccine is yet available against HCV.[2]

Worldwide Prevalence and Disease Burden

Recent analyses suggest that the global prevalence of chronic HCV (those who are HCV RNA positive) may be lower than previously projected. A systematic review in 2013, which included studies from 1980–2007 and utilized improved statistical modeling, projected the global prevalence of anti-HCV seroprevalence in 2005 to be 2.8% or 185 million individuals, of whom 130–150 million have chronic HCV.[3,4] However, another systematic review, which only included studies published in 2000 or later, estimated that the total global prevalence of anti-HCV seroprevalence was 1.6% or 115 million and that 80 million individuals were chronically infected.[5] These lower prevalence estimates may be due to increased mortality of the infected population as it ages and improved diagnostic tests with fewer false-positive results; but then, these may not reflect the more recent trends of increasing incidence of acute HCV in various parts of the world.[5–7]

The prevalence of chronic HCV infection is highest in West Sub-Saharan Africa (4.1% or 14.9 million), Central Sub-Saharan Africa (2.6% or 2.6 million), Eastern Europe (2.3% or 4.7 million), Central Asia (2.3% or 1.9 million), and North Africa/Middle East (2.1% or 9.7 million) as compared to North America (0.8% or 2.8 million) and Western Europe (0.6% or 2.6 million) (Table 2.1 and Figure 2.1).[5] Furthermore, 31 countries account for 80% of total infections, with China, Pakistan, Nigeria, Egypt, India, and Russia together contributing to greater than 50% of the total infections.

These estimates of global prevalence exclude high-risk populations, such as intravenous drug users, hemodialysis patients, and paid blood donors, who are not typically reflective of the general population. It is estimated that 67% of intravenous drug users worldwide are seropositive for anti-HCV (~10 million individuals); China (1.6 million), the United States (1.5 million), and Russia (1.3 million) have the largest HCV-exposed intravenous drug user populations.[8] Furthermore, the seroprevalence of HCV antibodies in patients on hemodialysis is estimated to be less than 5% in Northern Europe, approximately 10% in Southern Europe and the United States, and 10–68% in Asian, Latin American, and North African countries.[9]

The incidence of acute infection had previously declined as a result of screening of blood products and institution of universal precautions in medical settings[10] but since the late 2000s, there has been an increasing incidence of acute hepatitis C in various parts of the world, with most cases due to high-risk injection practices.[5–7] In addition, the burden of chronic HCV is increasing with time as the infected population ages. In fact, the Global Burden of Disease study reported an increase in the annual number of deaths due to HCV worldwide from 330,000 in 1990 to 704,000 in 2013.[11] Also, HCV is reported to be the cause of 27% of cirrhosis cases and 25% of HCC worldwide.[12]

Genotypes

HCV exhibits an extremely high degree of genetic diversity. There are seven main HCV genotypes (genotype 1 to 7), 67 confirmed and 20 provisional subtypes (a, b, c, etc.), and about 100 different strains (1, 2, 3, etc.) that differ at less than 15% of nucleotide sites.[13–15] The impact of viral genotypes in the pathogenesis of liver disease remains a subject of controversy, but the influence of the genotype in the response to specific direct-acting antiviral therapies or potential vaccines is well established. Thus, efforts to eradicate HCV through therapies and vaccine development necessitate a strong understanding of its global genotype distribution.

Genotypes 1–3 are widely distributed across the globe, whereas genotypes 4–6 are endemic to smaller regions (Figure 2.2). Genotype 1 accounts for 46% of HCV infections worldwide. Genotype 1a is predominantly located in Northern Europe, North America, and Australia, while genotype 1b is predominantly found in Southern and Eastern Europe, East Asia, and Japan. Genotype 3 is the next most common, accounting for 30% of cases globally and dominating in South Asia and parts of Scandinavia. Genotype 2 accounts

Table 2.1 Estimated prevalence of HCV seroprevalence and chronic infection by Global Burden of Disease regions

Region	Anti-HCV Prevalence (%)	Viremic HCV Prevalence (%)	Viremic rate (%)	2013 population (millions)	Anti-HCV infection (millions)	Viremic HCV infected (millions)
Asia Pacific, high-income	1.1	0.8	74	182	2.0	1.5
Asia, Central	5.4	2.3	43	84	4.5	1.9
Asia, East	1.2	0.7	60	1434	16.6	10.0
Asia, South	1.1	0.9	81	1650	18.8	15.2
Asia, Southwest	1.0	0.7	63	635	6.6	4.2
Australasia	1.4	1.0	75	28	0.4	0.3
Caribbean	0.8	0.6	70	39	0.3	0.2
Europe, Central	1.3	1.0	80	119	1.5	1.2
Europe, Eastern	3.3	2.3	69	207	6.8	4.7
Europe, Western	0.9	0.6	70	425	3.7	2.6
Latin America, Andean	0.9	0.6	70	57	0.5	0.4
Latin America, Central	1.0	0.8	75	246	2.6	1.9
Latin America, Southern	1.2	0.9	79	62	0.8	0.6
Latin America, Tropical	1.2	1.0	80	207	2.5	2.0
North Africa/Middle East	3.1	2.1	66	469	14.6	9.7
North America, high income	1.0	0.8	76	355	3.7	2.8
Oceania	0.1	0.1	69	10	0.0	0.0
Sub-Saharan Africa, Central	4.2	2.6	61	100	4.3	2.6
Sub-Saharan Africa, East	1.0	0.6	62	385	3.9	2.4
Sub-Saharan Africa, Southern	1.3	0.9	69	75	1.0	0.7
Sub-Saharan Africa, West	5.3	4.1	77	367	19.3	14.9
Other	1.9	1.3	69	27	0.5	0.4
Total	**1.6**	**1.1**	**70**	**7162**	**114.9**	**80.2**

Adapted from Gower E, Estes C, Blach S, Razavi-Shearer K, Razavi H. Global epidemiology and genotype distribution of the hepatitis C virus infection. *J Hepatol.* 2014;61(1):S45–57.

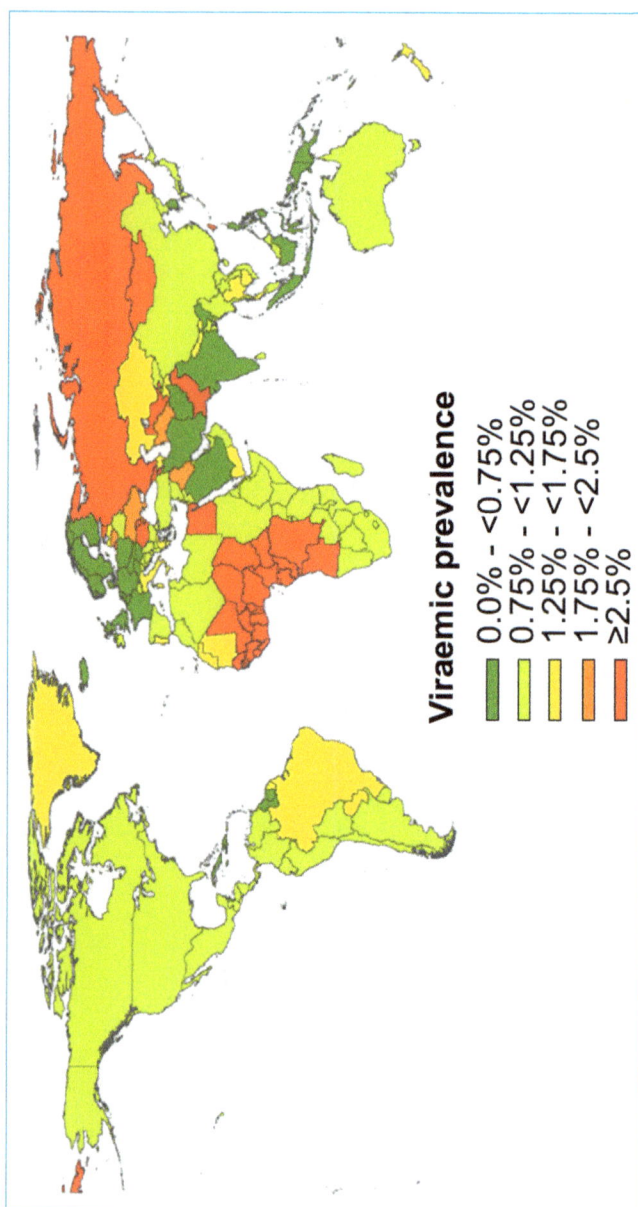

Figure 2.1 The prevalence of adult individuals with chronic HCV infection worldwide

Reproduced with permission from Gower E, Estes C, Blach S, Razavi-Shearer K, Razavi H. Global epidemiology and genotype distribution of the hepatitis C virus infection. *J Hepatol*. 2014;61(1):S45–57.

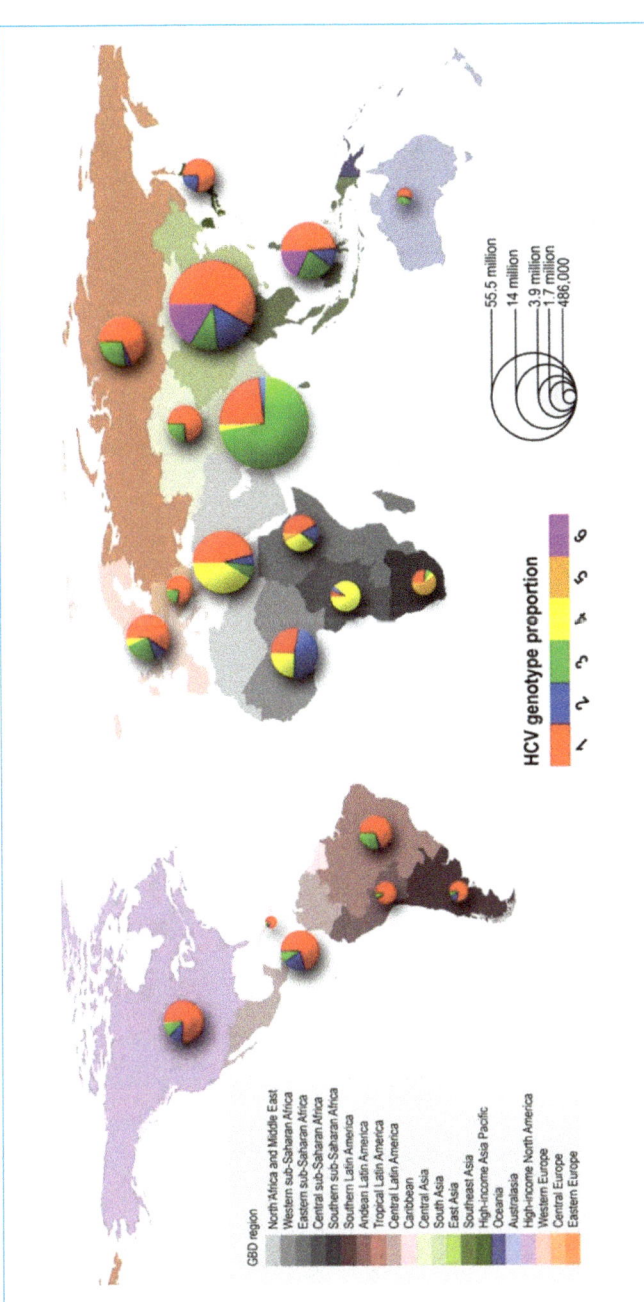

Figure 2.2 The relative prevalence of each HCV genotype by GBD region. Size of pie charts is proportional to number of seroprevalent cases as estimated by Hanafiah et al[3]

Reproduced with permission from Messina JP, Humphreys I, Flaxman A, et al. Global Distribution and Prevalence of Hepatitis C Virus Genotypes. *Hepatology*. 2015;6.

for 9% of cases worldwide and is found mostly in West Africa and East Asia. Genotype 4 is responsible for 8% of the global burden of HCV and is characteristic for the Middle East and North and Central Africa, including Egypt. Genotype 6 is the next most common, accounting for 5%, and dominates in South-East Asia. Genotype 5 is responsible for the fewest HCV cases globally (<1%) and is almost exclusively found in South Africa and Eastern Sub-Saharan Africa (Figure 2.2).[5,14] Genotype 7 has only been isolated once, in Central African emigrants living in Canada.[16]

Epidemiology in the United States

In the United States, the prevalence of HCV infection has been estimated from the National Health and Nutrition Examination Survey (NHANES). NHANES III data gathered from 1988 to 1994 estimated that 1.8% of the US population or 3.9 million individuals were exposed to hepatitis C as detected by serum HCV antibody and that 74% of exposed or 2.7 million individuals harbored the virus chronically.[17] An analysis of NHANES data from 1999 to 2002 reported a similar overall prevalence of HCV exposure at 1.6% or 4.1 million individuals and an estimated prevalence of chronic infection at 1.3% or 3.2 million individuals.[18] A more recent analysis of NHANES data from 2003 to 2010 estimated a similar prevalence of HCV exposure (1.3% or 3.6 million persons) and a prevalence of HCV RNA of 1.0% or 2.7 million persons.[19] The infection is more common in men (1.7%) than women (1.0%) and in non-Hispanic blacks (2.7%) than in non-Hispanic whites (1.1%) and Hispanics (0.8%). It is present in 0.1% of young individuals 20–29 years of age, peaks in prevalence at 3.2% in the 50- to 59-year age group, and decreases to 0.8% in persons who are 60 years or older. These findings represent an upward shift of the peak prevalence from the 35- to 39-year age group in the NHANES III study, as expected with aging of this group. Correspondingly, the estimated prevalence of chronic HCV infection among those born between 1945 and 1965 was 2.6% or 2.2 million persons.[19]

The survey, however, failed to assess several high-risk populations. Thus, it has been estimated that the true prevalence of chronic HCV infection in the United States is closer to 3.5–5.2 million when these groups are included.[20,21] HCV antibodies were detected in 32.1% (7.5–52.5%) of homeless persons tested, 15.6% (4.0–38.0%) of hospitalized patients, 4.5% (2.1–8.4%) of nursing home residents, 0.5% (0.48–0.84%) of active-duty military, and 11.5% (7.8–16.2%) of Native Americans living on reservations.[20,22,23] Furthermore, in 2012, there were 2.2 million individuals incarcerated in the United States.[24] These individuals have a high prevalence of HCV exposure, with a weighted mean estimate of 23% (7.5–44.0%).[20] About 30% of HCV-infected individuals spend time in a correctional facility, and IVDU was the most common risk factor. Interestingly, female inmates had higher prevalence rates than males, contrary to the general HCV-infected population, and this may be due to the higher rate of women being incarcerated for behaviors that are associated with increased risk for HCV, such as IVDU and prostitution.[25]

In the United States, genotype 1 predominates in 72.5% of the viremic individuals (46% for genotype 1a and 26% for genotype 1b). Genotype 2 was detected in 11% of persons with chronic HCV, genotype 3 in 9%, genotype 4 in 6%, and genotype 6 in 1%.[5] A similar distribution was reported by Messina and colleagues, with genotype 1 detected in 75% of Americans, genotype 2 in 12%, genotype 3 in 10%, genotype 4 in 1%, and genotypes 5 and 6 in less than 1%.[14]

Prior to the implementation of universal screening of blood donors in 1992, the predominant mode of transmission in the general HCV-infected population was exposure to infected blood and blood products. The enhanced screening of blood products led to a decline of the estimated incidence of acute hepatitis C from 180,000 in the mid-1980s to a nadir of 16,500 in 2011.[26] However, the number of new annual HCV infections increased significantly in 2014 to 30,500, which has been attributed to increasing rates of IVDU in young persons of less than 30 years of age from nonurban areas, especially east of the Mississippi River.[6,7]

As a result of the peak incidence in the late 1980s and early 1990s, the American population includes a substantial cohort of asymptomatic patients who are approaching the age at which the morbidity and mortality from HCV will begin to develop. In fact, the death rate from HCV had increased to 5.0 deaths/100,000 individuals in 2014, and the incidence of end-stage liver disease from HCV is predicted to quadruple in the next 20 years.[27] Moreover, at least 50% of individuals with chronic HCV are unaware of their diagnosis, including the populations at highest risk (Box 2.1).[28] The main impediment to the prevention and control of this growing burden of HCV is lack of knowledge and awareness about this disease among health care and social service providers, the lay community, and policy-makers[29] and inadequate access to effective therapy. Therefore, widespread understanding of the significant global and national burden of chronic HCV and removal of various barriers to therapy are needed to successfully eradicate the virus and its consequent impact on health.

Box 2.1 Who Should Be Tested for HCV Infection?

Persons born from 1945 through 1965
Persons who have ever injected illegal drugs, including those who have injected only once many years ago
Recipients of clotting factor concentrates made before 1987
Recipients of blood products or solid organ transplants before 1992
Patients who have ever received long-term hemodialysis therapy
Persons such as health care workers with known exposures to HCV, such as needlesticks
Recipients of blood products or organs from a donor who later tested positive for HCV
All HIV-infected persons
Patients with signs or symptoms of liver disease (e.g., abnormal liver enzyme tests)
Children born to HCV-infected mothers (HCV antibody should be tested after 18 months to avoid detecting maternal antibody)

Adapted from the US CDC, Hepatitis C Information for Health Professionals. Available at: http://www.cdc.gov/hepatitis/HCV/HCVfaq.htm (Accessed on January 12, 2017).

References

1. Centers for Disease Control and Prevention. Recommendations for Prevention and Control of Hepatitis C Virus (HCV) Infection and HCV-Related Chronic Disease. *MMWR*. 1998;47.

2. WHO. Hepatitis C, WHO Fact Sheet No. 164. Revised July 2016. Available from: http://www.who.int/mediacentre/factsheets/fs164/en/. Accessed on January 6, 2017.

3. Mohd Hanafiah K, Groeger J, Flaxman AD, Wiersma ST. Global epidemiology of hepatitis C virus infection: new estimates of age-specific antibody to HCV seroprevalence. *Hepatology*. 2013 Apr 1;57(4):1333–1342.

4. WHO. Guidelines for the screening, care and treatment of persons with chronic hepatitis C infection. Revised April 2016. Available from: http://www.who.int/hepatitis/publications/hepatitis-c-guidelines-2016/en/. Accessed on January 9, 2017.

5. Gower E, Estes C, Blach S, Razavi-Shearer K, Razavi H. Global epidemiology and genotype distribution of the hepatitis C virus infection. *J Hepatol*. 2014 Nov 1;61(1):S45–S57.

6. CDC. U.S. 2014 Surveillance Data for Viral Hepatitis. Revised September 2016. Available from: https://www.cdc.gov/hepatitis/statistics/2014surveillance/index.htm. Accessed on January 6, 2017.

7. Zibbell J, Iqbal K, Patel R, et al. Increases in hepatitis C virus infection related to injection drug use among persons aged ≤30 years: Kentucky, Tennessee, Virginia, and West Virginia, 2006–2012. *MMWR*. 2015 May 8;64(17):453–458.

8. Nelson P, Mathers B, Cowie B, et al. The epidemiology of viral hepatitis among people who inject drugs: results of global systematic reviews. *Lancet*. 2011 Aug 13;378(9791):571–583.

9. Kidney Disease: Improving Global Outcomes (KDIGO). KDIGO clinical practice guidelines for the prevention, diagnosis, evaluation, and treatment of hepatitis C in chronic kidney disease. *Kidney Int Suppl*. 2008 Apr;109:S1–S99.

10. EASL International Consensus Conference on Hepatitis C Paris, 26–28 February 1999. *J Hepatol*. 1999 May 1;30(5):956–9561.

11. GBD 2013 Mortality and Causes of Death Collaborators. Global, regional, and national age–sex specific all-cause and cause-specific mortality for 240 causes of death, 1990–2013: a systematic analysis for the Global Burden of Disease Study 2013. *Lancet*. 2015 Jan 16;385(9963):117–171.

12. Perz JF, Armstrong GL, Farrington LA, et al. The contributions of hepatitis B virus and hepatitis C virus infections to cirrhosis and primary liver cancer worldwide. *J Hepatol*. 2006 Oct;45(4):529–538.

13. Smith DB, Bukh J, Kuiken C, et al. Expanded classification of hepatitis C virus into 7 genotypes and 67 subtypes: updated criteria and genotype assignment web resource. *Hepatology*. 2014 Jan;59(1):318–327.

14. Messina JP, Humphreys I, Flaxman A, et al. Global distribution and prevalence of hepatitis C virus genotypes. *Hepatology*. 2015 Jan;61(1):77–87.

15. Global surveillance and control of hepatitis C. *J Viral Hepat*. 1999 Jan 1;6(1):35–47.

16. Murphy DG, Willems B, Deschênes M, et al. Use of sequence analysis of the NS5B region for routine genotyping of hepatitis C virus with reference to C/E1 and 5′ untranslated region sequences. *J Clin Microbiol*. 2007 Apr;45(4):1102–1112.

17. Alter MJ, Kruszon-Moran D, Nainan OV, et al. The prevalence of hepatitis C virus infection in the United States, 1988 through 1994. *N Engl J Med*. 1999 Aug 19;341(8):556–562.

18. Armstrong GL. The prevalence of hepatitis C virus infection in the United States, 1999 through 2002. *Ann Intern Med*. 2006 May 16;144(10):705.

19. Denniston MM, Jiles RB, Drobeniuc J, et al. Chronic hepatitis C virus infection in the United States, National Health and Nutrition Examination Survey 2003 to 2010. *Ann Intern Med*. 2014 Mar 4;160(5):293–300.

20. Edlin BR, Eckhardt BJ, Shu MA, et al. Toward a more accurate estimate of the prevalence of hepatitis C in the United States. *Hepatology*. 2015 Nov;62(5):1353–1363.

21. Chak E, Talal AH, Sherman KE, et al. Hepatitis C virus infection in USA: an estimate of true prevalence. *Liver Int*. 2011 Sep 1;31(8):1090–1101.

22. Chien NT, Dundoo G, Horani MH, et al. Seroprevalence of viral hepatitis in an older nursing home population. *J Am Geriatr Soc*. 1999 Sep;47(9):1110–1113.

23. Neumeister AS, Pilcher LE, Erickson JM, et al. Hepatitis-C prevalence in an urban native-American clinic: a prospective screening study. *J Natl Med Assoc*. 2007 Apr;99(4):389–392.

24. Bureau of Justice Statistics (BJS). Correctional Populations in the United States, 2012. Revised December 2013. Available from: https://www.bjs.gov/index.cfm?ty=pbse&sid=5. Accessed on January 12, 2017.

25. Vescio MF, Longo B, Babudieri S, et al. Correlates of hepatitis C virus seropositivity in prison inmates: a meta-analysis. *J Epidemiol Community Health*. 2008 Apr 1;62(4):305–313.

26. CDC. U.S. 2011 Surveillance Data for Viral Hepatitis. Revised August 2013. Available from: https://www.cdc.gov/hepatitis/statistics/2011surveillance/index.htm. Accessed on January 12, 2017.

27. Rein DB, Wittenborn JS, Weinbaum CM, et al. Forecasting the morbidity and mortality associated with prevalent cases of pre-cirrhotic chronic hepatitis C in the United States. *Dig Liver Dis*. 2011 Jan;43(1):66–72.

28. Yehia BR, Schranz AJ, Umscheid CA, Iii VLR. The treatment cascade for chronic hepatitis C virus infection in the United States: a systematic review and meta-analysis. *Plos One*. 2014 Jul 2;9(7):e101554.

29. Mitchell AE, Colvin HM, Palmer Beasley R. Institute of Medicine recommendations for the prevention and control of hepatitis B and C. *Hepatology*. 2010 Mar 1;51(3):729–733.

Chapter 3

Natural History of Hepatitis C

Cassandra Fritz and Andrew Aronsohn

Introduction

Hepatitis C virus (HCV) is the most common cause of death from liver disease and the leading cause for liver transplantation in the United States.[1-3] This chapter reviews the natural history of hepatitis C, from transmission to the development of chronic liver disease and its associated complications.

Risk Factors for Transmission

The dominant risks for hepatitis C transmission are intravenous drug use (IVDU), blood, and blood product transfusions. Hepatitis C is less commonly transmitted through sexual intercourse, intranasal drug use, and vertical transmission by HCV-infected mothers and health care–related exposures (Figure 3.1). Individuals with repeated direct percutaneous exposures or those with large-volume exposures have a higher prevalence of HCV, while those with infrequent small-volume exposures or mucosal contact have much lower prevalence rates (Figure 3.2).

Illicit Drug and Other Behavioral Transmission

IVDU still accounts for approximately half of all cases of acute hepatitis C in the United States.[4,5] Although rates of IVDU and incidence of hepatitis C virus were decreasing until 2006, recent data support an emerging epidemic of HCV infection in predominately white nonurban persons less than 30 years old.[6,7] The prevalence of HCV among patients who use IV drugs ranges from 27% to 93%.[8] This wide range of HCV prevalence is primarily due to higher risk of infection with increased duration of drug use.[8,9] Risk of HCV is highest among those who have greater than 5 years of IVDU, those with daily IVDU, and those who inject both heroin and cocaine.[10] HCV can also be transmitted through intranasal cocaine use and shared paraphernalia. When proper hygienic techniques are not employed, HCV can be transmitted through cosmetic procedures such as piercings and tattoos, as well as through complementary treatments such as acupuncture. Recent studies have supported the notion that commercial tattoos and piercings have a low to relatively nonexistent risk, whereas noncommercial applications carry the majority of the risk in these categories.[11]

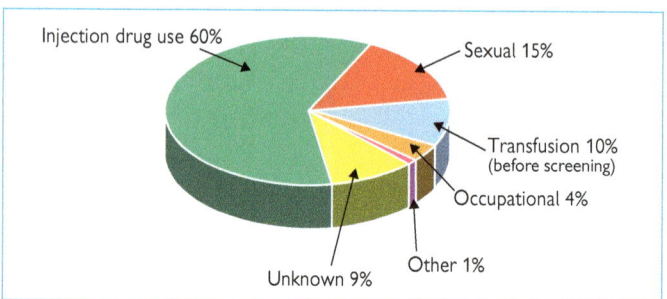

Figure 3.1 Sources of infection for persons with viral hepatitis C
Source: http://www.chronicliverdisease.org/library/slide/slide_topic.cfm?topic=ed3_epidemiology, Slide 13

Sexual Transmission

Although sexual transmission of HCV does occur, the virus is transmitted inefficiently through sexual contact, and the rate of transmission among long-term sexual partners is low. The seroconversion rate among monogamous heterosexual partners where one person is infected is less than 1% annually.[12] The prevalence of hepatitis C among spouses of HCV-positive persons is 1.5% to 5%, though shared high-risk behaviors may also contribute to this number.[13,14] Due to the low rate of transmission among monogamous partners, the US Centers for Disease Control (CDC) does not specifically recommend initiating barrier protection among monogamous partners. Household members should avoid sharing razors, toothbrushes, or other items that could lead to percutaneous exposure to blood.[13]

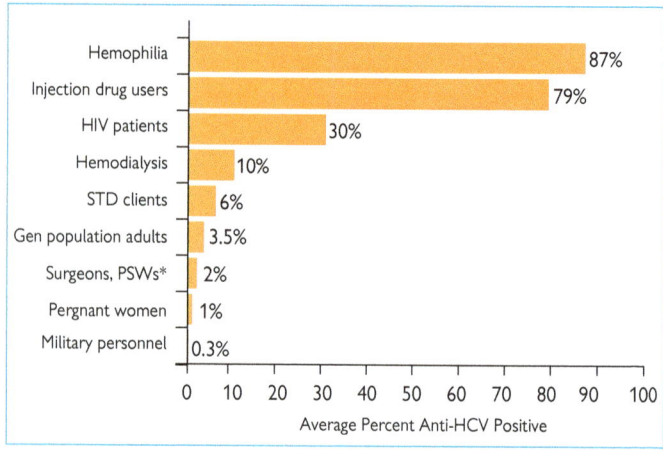

Figure 3.2 HCV prevalence by selected groups in the United States
Source: http://www.chronicliverdisease.org/library/slide/slide_topic.cfm?topic=ed3_epidemiology, Slide 14

Persons with high-risk sexual behaviors such as unprotected sex and more than 20 lifetime sexual partners have higher rates of hepatitis C.[15] In addition, risk of sexual transmission may be increased in the setting of acute HCV infection due to high viral concentrations and minimal antibody complexes.[16]

HIV-infected men who have sex with men (MSM), especially those who engage in sexual behaviors that increase mucosal trauma, are also at increased risk for infection with hepatitis C.[17,18] In this population, HCV prevalence has increased from 5.6% in 1995 to 20.9% in 2008.[19] The prevalence of HCV within the MSM HIV-negative population is similar to that found within the general population.[19,20] A low prevalence (1.5%) has also been reported in the MSM HIV-negative population who do not use intravenous drugs.[21]

Vertical Transmission

Maternal–fetal transmission, also known as vertical transmission, is thought to be the primary mode for transmission among children. Vertical transmission occurs almost exclusively in women with a detectable viral load. A meta-analysis examining maternal–fetal transmission rates found that the estimated risk for vertical transmission for HCV antibody-positive, HCV RNA-positive, and HIV-negative women is 5.8%, while HIV-positive woman have an infant transmission rate of 10.8%.[22] The increased transmission rate noted among coinfected mothers is thought to be due to increased hepatitis C viral load.[22] The timing and mode of transmission from mother to child remain unclear. Data from one prospective cohort study suggest that at least one-third of infected infants acquired infection in utero, with intrapartum and peripartum infection accounting for other infections.[23] Prolonged rupture of membranes, vaginal lacerations, and procedures that expose the fetus to maternal blood, such as fetal scalp monitors, all may increase the risk of transmission. Moreover, vertical transmission appears to increase when women have high ALT levels the year leading up to pregnancy through delivery.[24]

HCV antibody-positive pregnant women have significantly higher rates of cholestasis of pregnancy, preterm delivery, premature rupture of membranes, placental abruption, low birth weight, and overall perinatal mortality.[24] Pregnancy may worsen HCV-associated liver injury and necrosis; however, the long-term clinical significance of this type of injury is unknown.[25]

Current recommendations are to only screen pregnant women with risk factors for HCV. However, there has been some interest in instituting universal screening of women considering pregnancy now that HCV has an effective and safe cure.[26] Few measures can be taken to reduce the risk of vertical transmission of HCV, especially since treatment of HCV is currently contraindicated during pregnancy. Delivery by elective cesarean section has not been shown to reduce the rate of infection.[27] HCV is not transmitted through nursing, despite low levels of HCV present in milk, and therefore infected women may breastfeed in the absence of skin or nipple breakdown that would expose the infant to blood.[28] All infants born to HCV-infected mothers should be tested for HCV RNA on two separate occasions, between 2 and 6 months and at 18 to 24 months.[16]

Nosocomial Transmission

While blood transfusion was identified as a likely source of infection in 15% of acute hepatitis C cases in 1982, subsequent improvements in donor and blood screening techniques have reduced the risk greatly. In the 1960s,

20% of patients receiving transfusion experienced a posttransfusion hepatitis, of which the vast majority of cases were non-A/non-B hepatitis, later identified as hepatitis C. Changes in donor screening were initiated in 1978, including the transition to a volunteer-only donor pool and the addition of donor exclusion criteria, thus decreasing the risk of posttransfusion hepatitis. Universal testing for anti-HCV was initiated in 1990, and blood transfusions have accounted for less than 2% of HCV infections after 1992. The addition of nucleic acid testing for HCV in 1999 further decreased the risk of acquiring hepatitis C from blood transfusion, which is currently estimated at only 1 in 2 million units transfused. Persons with hemophilia who received concentrated clotting factors prior to 1989 had a greater than 90% prevalence of HCV.[13] Beginning in 1989, viral inactivation procedures were initiated, dramatically decreasing the risk of viral exposure. Still, the prevalence of HCV in this population remains high due to the chronicity of disease.

Although HCV health-related epidemics have been reported to be rare, nosocomial HCV transmissions have increased in recent years. The CDC investigated more than 33 HCV-related health care outbreaks from 1998 to 2012.[29] Most outbreaks are due to failure to comply with recommended sterilization techniques, including improper reuse of syringes and multiuse medication vials, in addition to improperly cleaned environmental surfaces at dialysis centers.[30] The risk of HCV transmission to a health care provider has been reported as a wide range of 0–10% after a needlestick injury from an infected patient. Yet a prospective 10-year study reported only a 1.8% seroconversion rate among health care workers after needlestick exposure.[31] HCV seroconversion may be further increased when the patient's viral load exceeds 500,000.[32]

Host Response to HCV

Acute Hepatitis C

Only 15–30% of people who acquire hepatitis C virus will develop clinically recognizable acute hepatitis C, manifested by acute onset of malaise, jaundice, influenza-like symptoms, elevated aminotransferase levels, and serologic evidence of hepatitis C infection.[4] Symptom onset occurs within 5–12 weeks after exposure and lasts anywhere between 2 and 12 weeks.[33] Yet, since the majority of acute infections are believed to be asymptomatic, HCV is infrequently diagnosed during the acute exposure.[33] Fulminant hepatitis C is exceedingly rare, and mortality among those with acute hepatitis C is less than 1% (Table 3.1).[4]

Testing and Serologies

Hepatitis C RNA is detectable by assays as early as 2 weeks after exposure to the virus, while anti-HCV does not become detectable until approximately 8–12 weeks after exposure.[34] Thus, screening using anti-HCV only may not detect those who have acquired HCV infection within the previous 8–12 weeks, also known as a "window period." Individuals who clear hepatitis C virus will have undetectable HCV RNA but will remain anti-HCV positive. Individuals with positive HCV RNA and anti- HCV in the absence of an

Table 3.1 Features of hepatitis C virus infection

HCA RNA first detected in blood	1–3 weeks
Time until symptoms (if any)	Average 6–7 weeks
	Range 2–26 weeks
Antibody first detected in blood	In 50–70% at onset of symptoms; in 90% by 3 months
Acute illness (jaundice)	Mild (≤ 20%)
Chronic infection (mostly asx)	75%–85%
Cirrhosis	10%–20%
Mortality from CLD	1%–5%

Source: http://www.chronicliverdisease.org/library/slide/slide_topic.cfm?topic=ed3_epidemiology, Slide 35.

acute infection or with anti-HCV and HCV RNA persistent for more than 6 months after the acute infection meet the criteria for chronic hepatitis C (Figure 3.3A, B).

Factors Affecting Spontaneous Clearance of the Virus

Acute HCV infection is followed by spontaneous clearance in only 20–25% of infections.[35,36] The remaining 75% of patients with acute hepatitis C infection will develop chronic hepatitis C (CHC), although certain populations have higher rates of spontaneous clearance of the virus. Specifically, women and children appear to have higher rates of clearance. An Irish study investigating young women with hepatitis C exposures from contaminated anti-D immunoglobulin demonstrated a clearance rate of 45%.[37] Similarly, 45% of children infected with hepatitis C after perioperative blood transfusions spontaneously cleared the virus.[38] Jaundice, though present in less than 10% of infections, is a clinical marker for a robust host immune response and is associated with a higher rate of spontaneous clearance of the virus.[34,39] Genome-wide association studies have identified rs12979860 (CC) polymorphism, located 3 kb upstream from the *IL28b* gene, as an important predictor of response to standard interferon therapy and spontaneous clearance (SC) of HCV. *IL28b* encodes interferon (IFN)-λ3, whose role in controlling the virus is unknown.[40] *IL28b* has been shown to be an important predictor of viral clearance among infants with perinatal exposures to hepatitis C.[41] The single nucleotide polymorphisms (SNPs) rs 12979860 (C/C) and rs8099917 (T/T)[36] appear to play a significant role in overall spontaneous clearance, with the C/C polymorphism being three times more likely to spontaneously clear the virus than those with the T/T polymorphism.[42] Although the *IL28b* genotype has been shown to be an important factor in SC, it is important to note that the majority of these studies have been conduced in predominately Caucasian and Asian populations. *IL28b* is not the only factor to determine SC; ethnicity, HCV genotype, stage of fibrosis,[36] and abstinence from alcohol in women[43] have also been shown to have a significant role. More recently, *IL-6* and *HLA-DQB1* have been associated with SC of HCV.[44]

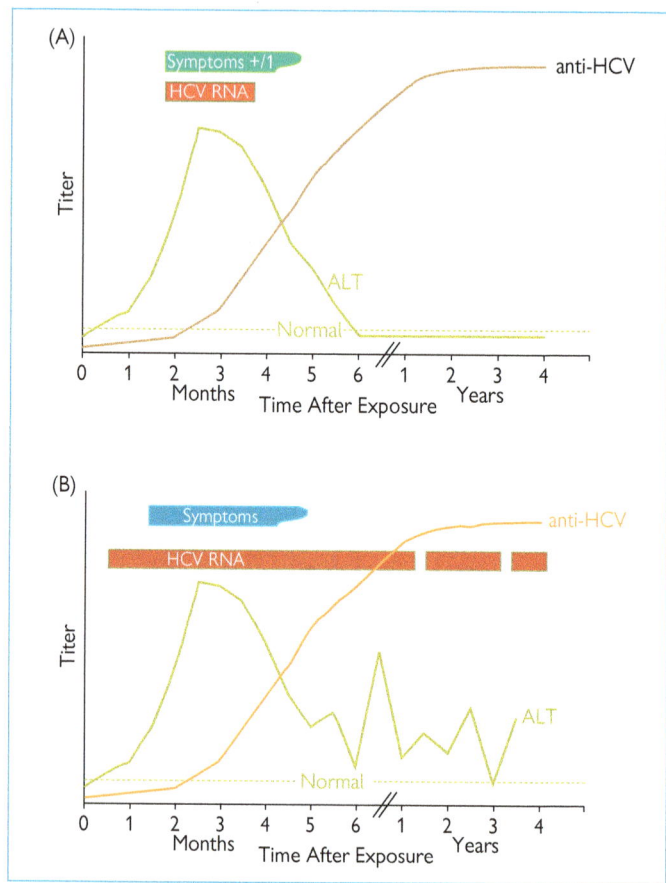

Figure 3.3 A and B serologic pattern of acute HCV infection in recovery (A) and with progression to chronic infection (B)

Source: http://www.chronicliverdisease.org/library/slide/slide_topic.cfm?topic=ed3_epidemiology, Slides 36; http://www.chronicliverdisease.org/library/slide/slide_topic.cfm?topic=ed3_epidemiology, Slides 37

Chronic Hepatitis C

Overall, 65–80% of people infected with hepatitis C will develop chronic disease.[15] Patients with CHC are often asymptomatic prior to developing cirrhosis or may exhibit symptoms such as fatigue, myalgias or arthralgias, weight loss, anorexia, and mental slowing. Extrahepatic manifestations of hepatitis C, such as cryoglobulinemia and porphyria cutanea tarda, are secondary to effects of the virus and can occur in the absence of liver disease. Although spontaneous clearance of chronic hepatitis C is exceedingly rare, female sex, younger age, lower HCV viral load, and hepatitis B surface antigen positivity have been associated with clearance.[45]

The rate of progression to cirrhosis varies from individual to individual but in general occurs over decades. Approximately 16% of patients

> **Box 3.1 Factors Associated with Accelerated Disease Progression**
>
> - HIV coinfection (immunosuppression)
> - Hepatitis B coinfection
> - Infection with HCV genotype 3
> - Older age at time of infection (age >40)
> - Male gender
> - Chronic alcohol consumption (>50 g/day)
> - Chronic daily marijuana use
> - Daily cigarette smoking
> - Obesity and insulin resistance
> - Diabetes
> - Hepatic steatosis
> - Genetic factors (under investigation)

develop cirrhosis at 20 years post infection, with 41% developing cirrhosis by 30 years.[46] Hepatic decompensation, including variceal bleeding, ascites, encephalopathy, and jaundice, occurs in one-third of patients with HCV cirrhosis for more than 10 years.[47] Five-year survival in those who have experienced some manifestation of hepatic decompensation is approximately 50% (Figure 3.5).[47]

Factors Affecting Disease Progression

Only 20–40% of those with CHC progress to cirrhosis. The variability in liver-related morbidity and mortality caused by HCV can be at least partially explained by host and viral factors that play a role in progression of hepatitis C to advanced liver disease (Box 3.1 and Figure 3.4).

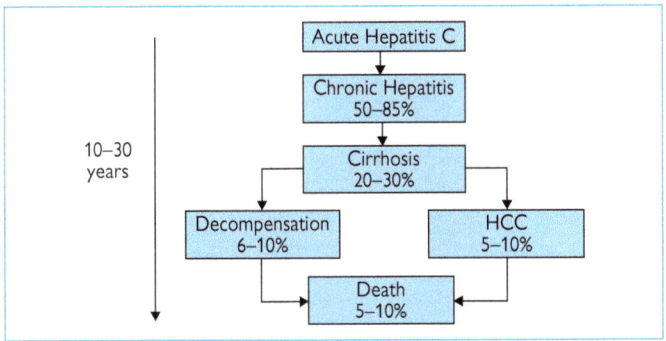

Figure 3.4 Natural history of hepatitis C
Source: http://www.chronicliverdisease.org/library/ slide/slide_topic.cfm?topic=ed3_epidemiology, Slide 39

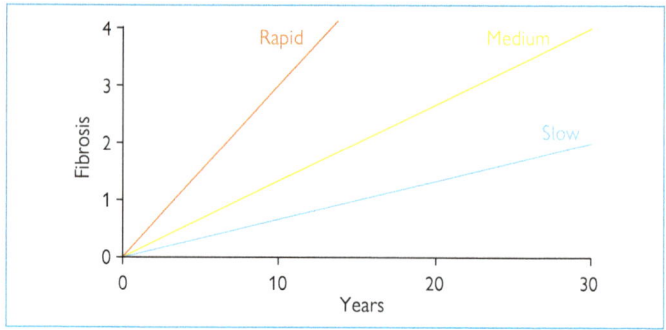

Figure 3.5 Modeling of liver fibrosis in HCV: different rates of progression
Source: http://www.chronicliverdisease.org/library/slide/slide_topic.cfm?topic=ed3_epidemiology, Slide 45

Fibrosis to Cirrhosis

Chronic HCV infection causes inflammation and injury resulting in fibrogenesis. Fibrosis is characterized by deposition of collagen and extracellular matrix proteins resulting in loss of liver architecture and, ultimately, cirrhosis. Biopsy is the gold standard for evaluating fibrosis, although noninvasive markers are also used to estimate the degree of fibrosis. Cross-sectional studies have shown that fibrosis progresses in a relatively linear fashion, with a median time to cirrhosis of 30 years. However, rates of progression to fibrosis are not normally distributed, with patients separating into groups of slow, intermediate, and rapid progressors (Figure 3.5).[48] Host and viral factors play a role in the rate of progression of disease and are discussed later. A systematic review concluded that the risk of developing HCV-related cirrhosis demonstrates an exponential relationship with duration of infection, as the estimated probability of cirrhosis is 16% at 20 years post exposure and 41% at 30 years post exposure.[46]

Demographic Factors

Age

Children and young women have been shown to have lower rates of progression to cirrhosis as well as increased rates of spontaneous viral clearance.[37,38] Alternatively, acquiring the disease at an older age (after age 40–50) is associated with an accelerated progression of liver injury.[48,49] Cross-sectional studies have shown age to be an independent predictor of fibrosis progression, and progression is most rapid in those infected after age 50.[48,50] Even among those infected at a younger age, cirrhosis progression is still accelerated after reaching age 50.[50] The mechanisms behind the increased progression are still not fully elucidated. The aging liver is less able to adapt to injury, and age-related changes in hepatocyte proliferation and response to oxidative stress have been noted.[51] Furthermore, aged persons demonstrate a significant decline in immune response, particularly in relation to T cells, and this host–virus interaction may also play a role.[52]

Race

African-Americans, despite having a higher liver-related mortality than whites, appear to have a slower rate of progression of fibrosis.[53–55] Data comparing progression among other races are not as robust, although progression appears to be accelerated in non-black American Hispanics as compared to whites.[56]

Behavioral Factors

Alcohol consumption in the setting of chronic HCV has been associated with a twofold increased risk of progression to cirrhosis and HCC and of overall mortality. Its use, even at moderate levels, is associated with increased HCV RNA levels and higher rates of fibrosis.[57–59] A safe amount of alcohol use has not been established for those with CHC; therefore, abstinence from alcohol is recommended. Chronic daily marijuana use and tobacco smoking have also been shown to increase the rate of progression of steatosis and fibrosis.[60]

Metabolic Factors

Metabolic factors, including obesity and insulin resistance, adversely affect outcomes in CHC. HCV has been strongly associated with metabolic derangements and steatosis as the prevalence of steatosis within this population is much higher.[61] This was demonstrated in patients with insulin resistance and evidence of baseline steatosis who were shown to be at increased risk of histologic progression of fibrosis and complications of cirrhosis.[62] Small studies have shown improvement in aminotransferase levels with weight loss among obese patients with chronic liver disease, suggesting that a weight loss program would be a reasonable intervention.[63] Furthermore, diabetes appears to be a poor prognostic factor in patients with CHC and cirrhosis.[64]

Coinfections

Patients who are coinfected with HIV have higher HCV RNA levels. HIV coinfection has been shown to accelerate progression of cirrhosis, liver failure, and HCC in HCV-infected individuals.[65] Up to one-fourth of patients with HIV are coinfected with hepatitis C due to overlapping risk factors and an impaired immune response that decreases clearance rates. A low CD4 count portends a fourfold relative risk of hepatic decompensation.[66] To date, there is no evidence that early initiation of highly active antiretroviral therapy (HAART) in coinfected patients delays progression.[66] Coinfection with HBV or with multiple strains of HCV also results in increased disease progression. Thus, abstaining from high-risk behaviors such as IVDU, even after acquiring chronic hepatitis C, is prudent.[56] Patients should be screened for HIV and hepatitis B at the time of diagnosis to allow for immunization of those who are not immune to HBV and consideration for HIV treatment.

Viral Factors

Although HCV genotype plays a crucial role in treatment outcomes, only genotype 3 is independently associated with increased progression of liver disease. However, it is also linked with increased steatosis independent from predisposing conditions, and it is hypothesized that the increased steatosis is the predominant reason for accelerated disease progression.[56] A large retrospective cohort study demonstrated that, when compared to genotype 1, patients with genotype 3 were 31% more likely to develop cirrhosis and 80% more likely to develop HCC.[67]

Genetic Factors

In a meta-analysis, *IL28b* polymorphisms appear to modify the natural disease progression of patients with CHC, and disease progression appears to be promoted in the CC and TT genotypes.[68] Various other target gene polymorphisms have been investigated including HLA classes, profibrogenic cytokines, PNPLA3,[69,70] let-7 microRNA,[71] and DEPDC5 genetic variants.[72] Although further investigation in the role of host genetics in disease progression is needed, one genome-wide association study identified seven SNPS that in combination were predictors of cirrhosis,[73] while another study has demonstrated that *IL-10* SNPs are associated with disease severity.[74] The majority of studies investigating genetic factors in HCV disease progression are limited to Caucasian and Asian patient populations.

Hepatocellular Carcinoma

Hepatitis C–related cirrhosis accounts for approximately one third of HCC cases in the United States. Almost all hepatitis C–related HCC is found in the setting of cirrhosis, in which the incidence is estimated to be between 2% and 8% per year.[75,76] Multiple factors are associated with HCV-related HCC: age greater than 60, alcohol consumption, obesity, and insulin resistance.[77,78] As medical care for end-stage liver disease improves and affected individuals live longer, HCC has become an important indication for liver transplantation.

CHC and Survival

Chronic HCV infection is associated with a 2.37-times higher mortality rate ratio than healthy controls and a 26-fold increase in liver-related mortality.[79] Interestingly, those with positive anti-HCV without CHC still had a 1.79-times higher mortality rate. Behavioral and lifestyle risks that predispose to HCV exposure may also contribute to non–liver-related mortality increase. Among a group of individuals with compensated cirrhosis, 5- and 10-year transplant-free survival rates were 91% and 79%, respectively.[76] Five-year survival after liver transplantation for CHC is relatively unchanged over the past two decades at approximately 72%.[80]

Conclusion

Chronic hepatitis C is a common cause of liver disease worldwide. As therapeutic interventions for CHC continue to improve, continued focus on the natural history of the disease will be a key component in reducing overall liver-related morbidity and mortality.

References

1. Ghany MG, Strader DB, Thomas DL, Seeff LB. Diagnosis, management, and treatment of hepatitis C: an update. *Hepatology.* 2009;49(4):1335–1374.
2. Smith BD, Jorgensen C, Zibbell JE, Beckett GA. Centers for Disease Control and Prevention initiatives to prevent hepatitis C virus infection: a selective update. *Clin Infect Dis.* 2012;55(suppl 1):S49–S53.
3. Sarpel D, Baichoo E, Dieterich DT. Chronic hepatitis B and C infection in the United States: a review of current guidelines, disease burden and cost effectiveness of screening. *Expert Rev Anti Infect Ther.* 2016;14(5):511–521.
4. Williams IT, Bell BP, Kuhnert W, Alter MJ. Incidence and transmission patterns of acute hepatitis C in the United States, 1982–2006. *Arch Intern Med.* 2011;171(3):242–248.
5. Ditah I, Ditah F, Devaki P, et al. The changing epidemiology of hepatitis C virus infection in the United States: national health and nutrition examination survey 2001 through 2010. *J Hepatol.* 2014;60(4):691–698.
6. Zibbell JE, Iqbal K, Patel RC, et al. Increases in hepatitis C virus infection related to injection drug use among persons aged≤ 30 years-Kentucky, Tennessee, Virginia, and West Virginia, 2006–2012. *MMWR.* 2015;64(17):453–458.
7. Suryaprasad AG, White JZ, Xu F, et al. Emerging epidemic of hepatitis C virus infections among young non-urban persons who inject drugs in the United States, 2006–2012. *Clin Infect Dis.* 2014;59(10):1411–1419.
8. Chak E, Talal AH, Sherman KE, Schiff ER, Saab S. Hepatitis C virus infection in USA: an estimate of true prevalence. *Liver Int.* 2011;31(8):1090–1101.
9. Tseng FC, O'Brien TR, Zhang M, Kral AH, Ortiz-Conde BA, Lorvick J, Busch M, Edlin BR. Seroprevalence of hepatitis C virus and hepatitis B virus among San Francisco injection drug users, 1998 to 2000. *Hepatology.* 2007;46(3):666–671.
10. Amon JJ, Garfein RS, Ahdieh-Grant L, et al. Prevalence of hepatitis C virus infection among injection drug users in the United States, 1994–2004. *Clin Infect Dis.* 2008;46(12):1852–1858.
11. Klevens RM, Hu DJ, Jiles R, Holmberg SD. Evolving epidemiology of hepatitis C virus in the United States. *Clin Infect Dis.* 2012;55(suppl 1):S3–S9.
12. Tahan V, Karaca C, Yildirim B, et al. Sexual transmission of HCV between spouses. *Am J Gastroenterol.* 2005;100(4):821–824.
13. CDC. Recommendations for prevention and control of hepatitis C virus (HCV) infection and HCV-related chronic disease. *MMWR Recomm Rep.* 1998;47(RR-19):1–39.
14. Thomas DL, Zenilman JM, Alter HJ, et al. Sexual transmission of hepatitis C virus among patients attending sexually transmitted diseases clinics in Baltimore—an analysis of 309 sex partnerships. *J Infect Dis.* 1995;171(4):768–775.

15. Armstrong GL, Wasley A, Simard EP, McQuillan GM, Kuhnert WL, Alter MJ. The prevalence of hepatitis C virus infection in the United States, 1999 through 2002. *Ann Intern Med.* 2006;144(10):705–714.

16. Alter MJ. Epidemiology of hepatitis C virus infection. *World J Gastroenterol.* 2007;13(17):2436.

17. Sexual transmission of hepatitis C virus among HIV-infected men who have sex with men—New York City, 2005–2010. *MMWR.* 2011 July 22;60:945–950.

18. Taylor LE, Holubar M, Wu K, et al. Incident hepatitis C virus infection among US HIV-infected men enrolled in clinical trials. *Clin Infect Dis.* 2011;52(6), 812–818.

19. Urbanus AT, Van De Laar TJ, Geskus R, Vanhommerig JW, Van Rooijen MS, Schinkel J. Prins, M. Trends in hepatitis C virus infections among MSM attending a sexually transmitted infection clinic: 1995–2010. *AIDS.* 2014; 28(5):781–790.

20. Blaxhult A, Samuelson A, Ask R, Hökeberg I. Limited spread of hepatitis C among HIV-negative men who have sex with men in Stockholm, Sweden. *Int J STD AIDS.* 2013;25(7):493–495.

21. Buffington J, Murray PJ, Schlanger K, et al Low prevalence of hepatitis C virus antibody in men who have sex with men who do not inject drugs. *Public Health Rep.* 2007;122(Suppl 2):63.

22. Benova L, Mohamoud YA, Calvert C, Abu-Raddad LJ. Vertical transmission of hepatitis C virus: systematic review and meta-analysis. *Clin Infect Dis.* 2014;59(6):765–773.

23. Mok J, Pembrey L, Tovo PA, Newell ML. When does mother to child transmission of hepatitis C virus occur? *Arch Dis Child Fetal Neonatal Ed.* 2005;90(2):F156–F160.

24. Le Campion A, Larouche A, Fauteux-Daniel S, Soudeyns H. Pathogenesis of hepatitis C during pregnancy and childhood. *Viruses.* 2012;4(12):3531–3550.

25. Conte D, Fraquelli M, Prati D, Colucci A, Minola E. Prevalence and clinical course of chronic hepatitis C virus (HCV) infection and rate of HCV vertical transmission in a cohort of 15,250 pregnant women. *Hepatology.* 2000;31(3):751–755.

26. Aebi-Popp K, Duppenthaler A, Rauch A, et al. Vertical transmission of hepatitis C: towards universal antenatal screening in the era of new direct acting antivirals (DAAs)? Short review and analysis of the situation in Switzerland. *J Virus Erad.* 2016;2(1):52.

27. Ghamar Chehreh ME, Tabatabaei SV, Khazanehdari S, Alavian SM. Effect of cesarean section on the risk of perinatal transmission of hepatitis C virus from HCV-RNA+/HIV- mothers: a meta-analysis. *Arch Gynecol Obstet.* 2011;283(2):255–260.

28. Indolfi G, Resti M. Perinatal transmission of hepatitis C virus infection. *J Med Vriol.* 2009;81(5):836–843.

29. Ward JW. The epidemiology of chronic hepatitis C and one-time hepatitis C virus testing of persons born during 1945 to 1965 in the United States. *Clin Liver Dis.* 2013;17(1):1–11.

30. Thompson ND, Perz JF, Moorman AC, Holmberg SD. Nonhospital health care-associated hepatitis B and C virus transmission: United States, 1998–2008. *Ann Intern Med.* 2009;150(1):33–39.

31. Strasser M, Aigner E, Schmid I, Stadlmayr A, Niederseer D, Patsch W, Datz C. Risk of hepatitis C virus transmission from patients to healthcare workers: a prospective observational study. *Risk.* 2013;34(7):759–761.

32. Sulkowski MS, Ray SC, Thomas DL. Needlestick transmission of hepatitis C. *JAMA*. 2002;287(18):2406–2413.

33. Hajarizadeh B, Grebely J, Dore GJ. Epidemiology and natural history of HCV infection. *Nat Rev Gastroenterol Hepatol*. doi:10.1038/nrgastro.2013.107

34. Hofer H, Watkins-Riedel T, Janata O, et al. Spontaneous viral clearance in patients with acute hepatitis C can be predicted by repeated measurements of serum viral load. *Hepatology*. 2003;37(1):60–64.

35. Micallef JM, Kaldor JM, Dore GJ. Spontaneous viral clearance following acute hepatitis C infection: a systematic review of longitudinal studies. *J Viral Hepat*. 2006;13(1):34–41.

36. Jiménez-Sousa MA, Fernández-Rodríguez A, Guzmán-Fulgencio M, García-Álvarez M, Resino S. Meta-analysis: implications of interleukin-28B polymorphisms in spontaneous and treatment-related clearance for patients with hepatitis C. *BMC Med*. 2013;11(1):6.

37. Kenny-Walsh, E. Clinical outcomes after hepatitis C infection from contaminated anti-D immune globulin. Irish Hepatology Research Group. *N Engl J Med*. 1999;340(16):1228–1233.

38. Vogt M, Lang T, Frosner G, et al. Prevalence and clinical outcome of hepatitis C infection in children who underwent cardiac surgery before the implementation of blood-donor screening. *N Engl J Med*. 1999;341(12):866–870.

39. Maheshwari A, Ray S, Thuluvath PJ. Acute hepatitis C. *Lancet*. 2008;372(9635):321–332.

40. Marcello T, Grakoui A, Barba–Spaeth G, Machlin ES, Kotenko SV, Macdonald MR, Rice CM. Interferons α and λ inhibit hepatitis C virus replication with distinct signal transduction and gene regulation kinetics. *Gastroenterology*. 2006;131(6):1887–1898.

41. Ruiz-Extremera A, Munoz-Gamez JA, Salmeron-Ruiz MA, et al. Genetic variation in interleukin 28B with respect to vertical transmission of hepatitis C virus and spontaneous clearance in HCV-infected children. *Hepatology*. 2011;53(6):1830–1838.

42. Thomas DL, Thio CL, Martin MP, et al. Genetic variation in IL28B and spontaneous clearance of hepatitis C virus. *Nature*. 2009;461(7265):798–801.

43. Tsui JI, Mirzazadeh A, Hahn JA, et al. The effects of alcohol on spontaneous clearance of acute hepatitis C virus infection in females versus males. *Drug Alcohol Depend*. 2016;169:156–162.

44. Waldron PR, Belitskaya-Levy I, Chary A, et al. Genetic variation in the IL-6 and HLA-DQB1 genes is associated with spontaneous clearance of hepatitis C virus infection. *J Immunol Res*. 2016;2016;1–9.

45. Bulteel N, Sarathy PP, Forrest E, et al. Factors associated with spontaneous clearance of chronic hepatitis C virus infection. *J Hepatol*. 2016;65(2):266–272.

46. Thein HH, Yi Q, Dore GJ, Krahn MD. Estimation of stage-specific fibrosis progression rates in chronic hepatitis C virus infection: a meta-analysis and meta-regression. *Hepatology*. 2008;48(2):418–431.

47. Planas R, Balleste B, Alvarez MA, et al. Natural history of decompensated hepatitis C virus-related cirrhosis. A study of 200 patients. *J Hepatol*. 2004;40(5):823–830.

48. Poynard T, Bedossa P, Opolon P. Natural history of liver fibrosis progression in patients with chronic hepatitis C. The OBSVIRC, METAVIR, CLINIVIR, and DOSVIRC groups. *Lancet*. 1997;349(9055):825–832.

49. Seeff LB. Natural history of hepatitis C. *Hepatology*. 1997;26(3 Suppl 1):21S–28S.

50. Poynard T, Ratziu V, Charlotte F, Goodman Z, McHutchison J, Albrecht J. Rates and risk factors of liver fibrosis progression in patients with chronic hepatitis C. *J Hepatol.* 2001;34(5):730–739.

51. Hoare M, Das T, Alexander G. Ageing, telomeres, senescence, and liver injury. *J Hepatol.* 2010;53(5):950–961.

52. Solana R, Pawelec G. Molecular and cellular basis of immunosenescence. *Mech Ageing Dev.* 1998;102(2–3):115–129.

53. Crosse K, Umeadi OG, Anania FA, et al. Racial differences in liver inflammation and fibrosis related to chronic hepatitis C. *Clin Gastroenterol Hepatol.* 2004;2(6):463–468.

54. Sterling RK, Stravitz RT, Luketic VA, et al. A comparison of the spectrum of chronic hepatitis C virus between Caucasians and African Americans. *Clin Gastroenterol Hepatol.* 2004;2(6):469–473.

55. Wiley TE, Brown J, Chan J. Hepatitis C infection in African Americans: its natural history and histological progression. *Am J Gastroenterol.* 2002;97(3):700–706.

56. Missiha SB, Ostrowski M, Heathcote EJ. Disease progression in chronic hepatitis C: modifiable and nonmodifiable factors. *Gastroenterology.* 2008; 134(6):1699–1714.

57. Kyrlagkitsis I, Portmann B, Smith H, O'Grady J, Cramp ME. Liver histology and progression of fibrosis in individuals with chronic hepatitis C and persistently normal ALT. *Am J Gastroenterol.* 2003;98(7):1588–1593.

58. Martinot-Peignoux M, Boyer N, Cazals-Hatem D, et al. Prospective study on anti-hepatitis C virus-positive patients with persistently normal serum alanine transaminase with or without detectable serum hepatitis C virus RNA. *Hepatology.* 2001;34(5):1000–1005.

59. Puoti C, Castellacci R, Montagnese F, et al. Histological and virological features and follow-up of hepatitis C virus carriers with normal aminotransferase levels: the Italian prospective study of the asymptomatic C carriers (ISACC). *J Hepatol.* 2002;37(1):117–123.

60. Hezode C, Roudot-Thoraval F, Nguyen S, et al. Daily cannabis smoking as a risk factor for progression of fibrosis in chronic hepatitis C. *Hepatology.* 2005;42(1):63–71.

61. Lonardo A, Adinolfi LE, Restivo L, Ballestri S, Romagnoli D, Baldelli E, Loria P. Pathogenesis and significance of hepatitis C virus steatosis: an update on survival strategy of a successful pathogen. *World J Gastroenterol.* 2014;20(23):7089.

62. Everhart JE, Lok AS, Kim HY, et al. Weight-related effects on disease progression in the hepatitis C antiviral long-term treatment against cirrhosis trial. *Gastroenterology.* 2009;137(2):549–557.

63. Hickman IJ, Jonsson JR, Prins JB, et al. Modest weight loss and physical activity in overweight patients with chronic liver disease results in sustained improvements in alanine aminotransferase, fasting insulin, and quality of life. *Gut.* 2004;53(3):413–419.

64. Elkrief L, Chouinard P, Bendersky N, et al. Diabetes mellitus is an independent prognostic factor for major liver-related outcomes in patients with cirrhosis and chronic hepatitis C. *Hepatology.* 2014;60 (3):823–831.

65. Kang W, Tong HI, Sun Y, Lu Y. Hepatitis C virus infection in patients with HIV-1: epidemiology, natural history and management. *Exp Rev Gastroenterol Hepatol.* 2014;8(3):247–266.

66. Pineda JA, Garcia-Garcia JA, Aguilar-Guisado M, et al. Clinical progression of hepatitis C virus-related chronic liver disease in human immunodeficiency virus-infected patients undergoing highly active antiretroviral therapy. *Hepatology*. 2007;46(3):622–630.

67. Kanwal F, Kramer JR, Ilyas J, et al. HCV genotype 3 is associated with an increased risk of cirrhosis and hepatocellular cancer in a national sample of US Veterans with HCV. *Hepatology*. 2014;60(1):98–105.

68. Sato M, Kondo M, Tateishi R, Fujiwara N, Kato N, Yoshida H, Koike K. Impact of IL28B genetic variation on HCV-induced liver fibrosis, inflammation, and steatosis: a meta-analysis. *PloS One*. 2014;9(3):e91822.

69. Trepo E, Pradat P, Potthoff A, et al. Impact of patatin-like phospholipase-3 (rs738409 C>G) polymorphism on fibrosis progression and steatosis in chronic hepatitis C. *Hepatology*. 2011;54(1):60–69.

70. Nunez-Torres R, Macias J, Mancebo M, et al. The PNPLA3 genetic variant rs738409 influences the progression to cirrhosis in HIV/hepatitis C virus coinfected patients. *PloS One*. 2016;11(12):e0168265.

71. Matsuura K, De Giorgi VD, Schechterly C, et al. Circulating let-7 levels in plasma and extracellular vesicles correlate with hepatic fibrosis progression in chronic hepatitis C. *Hepatology*. 2016;64 (3):732–745.

72. Burza MA, Motta BM, Mancina RM, et al. DEPDC5 variants increase fibrosis progression in Europeans with chronic hepatitis C virus infection. *Hepatology*. 2016;63(2):418–427.

73. Huang H, Shiffman ML, Friedman S, et al. A 7 gene signature identifies the risk of developing cirrhosis in patients with chronic hepatitis C. *Hepatology*. 2007;46(2):297–306.

74. Świątek-Kościelna B, Kałużna E, Strauss E, et al. Interleukin 10 gene single nucleotide polymorphisms in Polish patients with chronic hepatitis C: analysis of association with severity of disease and treatment outcome. *Human Immunology*. 2017;78(2):192–200.

75. Degos F, Christidis C, Ganne-Carrie N, et al. Hepatitis C virus-related cirrhosis: time to occurrence of hepatocellular carcinoma and death. *Gut*. 2000;47(1):131–136.

76. Fattovich G, Giustina G, Degos F, et al. Morbidity and mortality in compensated cirrhosis type C: a retrospective follow-up study of 384 patients. *Gastroenterology*.1997;112(2):463–472.

77. Hamada H, Yatsuhashi H, Yano K, et al. Impact of aging on the development of hepatocellular carcinoma in patients with post transfusion chronic hepatitis C. *Cancer*. 2002;95(2):331–339.

78. Hassan MM, Hwang LY, Hatten CJ, et al. Risk factors for hepatocellular carcinoma: synergism of alcohol with viral hepatitis and diabetes mellitus. *Hepatology*. 2002;36(5):1206–1213.

79. El-Kamary SS, Jhaveri R, Shardell MD. All-cause, liver-related, and non-liver-related mortality among HCV-infected individuals in the general US population. *Clin Infect Dis*. 2011;53(2):150–157.

80. Watt KD, Burak KW, Deschenes M, et al. Survival after liver transplantation for hepatitis C is unchanged over two decades in Canada. *Can J Gastroenterol*. 2008;22(2):153.

Chapter 4

Diagnostic Testing for Hepatitis C

Natasha von Roenn

The initial evaluation for hepatitis C virus infection (HCV) encompasses both the decision to screen an individual for the disease and the evaluation that ensues once the diagnosis has been made. The diagnostic methods outlined in. Table 4.1 will be covered in this chapter.

Screening

Historically, the Centers for Disease Control and Prevention (CDC) and the American Association for the Study of Liver Diseases (AASLD) recommend focusing screening on individuals with risk factors for hepatitis C and those with an unexplained elevation in aminotransferase levels. Unfortunately, risk-based screening has failed to adequately identify most individuals with HCV. A recent proposal to the CDC's screening recommendations suggests that all individuals born between 1945 and 1965 get tested once for HCV. One-time cohort screening is estimated to identify nearly 86% of undiagnosed cases compared with the 21% currently found through risk-based screening.[1] These individuals are five times more likely to be infected with chronic HCV compared with other adults and currently account for more than 75% of infected individuals in the United States. Because HCV is often asymptomatic, it is critical that clinicians routinely take an appropriate history in order to identify risk factors, which should be done in combination with appropriate HCV testing and counseling.[2] The risk factors for hepatitis C were detailed in Chapter 3. For those who test positive during screening, the proposed CDC recommendations call for referral for treatment and a brief screening for alcohol use.

Antibody Testing

Detection of antibodies to HCV is the first step to screen patients in whom HCV is suspected. The presence of HCV antibodies is indicative of either past, current, or resolved infection and cannot discriminate between acute and chronic HCV infection. Antibodies may be detectable as early as 4–6 weeks after initial HCV exposure (Figure 4.1). Development of antibodies may be delayed, however, in patients who have subclinical infection.[3] Antibodies will persist indefinitely in chronically infected individuals, but

Table 4.1 Diagnostic testing used in patients with hepatitis C

Basic laboratory testing	Complete metabolic panel
	Complete blood count
	Prothrombin time
Serologic assays	Anti-HCV
	RIBA
Virologic assays	HCV RNA nucleic acid testing (NAT)
	Quantitative
	Qualitative
	HCV core antigen EIA assay
HCV genotyping with subtypes	1a-6
Liver biopsy	
Noninvasive markers of fibrosis	APRI
	FIBROSpect II
	FibroTest
	HepaScore
	Transient elastography
Genetic markers	IL28B

Source: © 2011 Natasha Walzer.

anti-HCV titers may decrease and even disappear in patients who clear HCV either spontaneously or after antiviral treatment.

The screening test is an enzyme immunoassay (EIA) that detects antibodies to recombinant antigens from core and nonstructural proteins that make up the HCV virion. EIA-2 (second-generation) testing detects HCV antibodies in

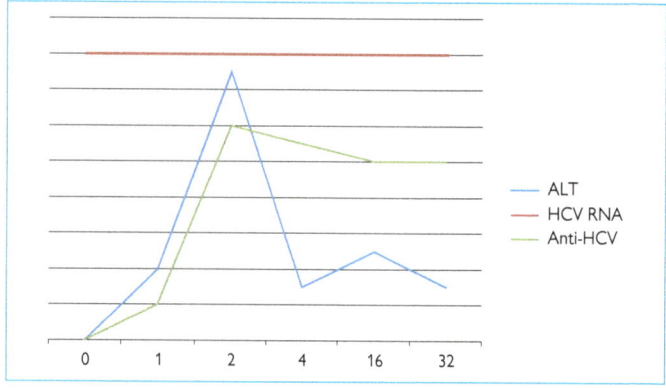

Figure 4.1 Serologic profile of chronic HCV infection The ALT will rise within the first month after acute infection and will fluctuate if the disease remains chronic. The HCV RNA will be the earliest detectable evidence for infection and remains fairly constant throughout the course of infection. Anti-HCV will be detectable within 4–6 weeks after infection and remains elevated even if there is clearance of the virus (either through treatment or spontaneously)

Source: © 2011 Natasha Walzer.

95% of infected individuals.[4] EIA-3 testing, which adds an additional antigen from the nonstructural region (NS5), has been introduced in many centers across the United States. When compared with second-generation assays, third-generation assays have sensitivities and specificities exceeding 99% and can detect HCV antibodies 2–3 weeks earlier.[5]

The sensitivity of EIAs appears to be reduced in immunocompromised persons, including those on hemodialysis, individuals infected with HIV, and transplant recipients.[6–8] Testing for HCV RNA should be considered in immunocompromised patients who are anti-HCV negative but have risk factors for HCV infection and persistently elevated aminotransferase levels.

An over-the-counter testing kit (Hepatitis C Check [Home Access Health Corp.]) has been approved by the US Food and Drug Administration (FDA). The blood sample is obtained at home using a lancet and shipped in a weather-resistant pouch. Upon arrival at the laboratory, standard EIAs are used to test the sample. The sensitivity of this method has been shown to be comparable to hospital-based laboratory testing. Pre- and posttest counseling is available through the manufacturer. In addition, a point-of-care test for rapid detection of anti-HCV was recently approved in Europe. It was shown to be as accurate as laboratory-based testing and could potentially increase access to HCV testing in the community.[9]

Confirmatory testing using recombinant immunoblot assay (RIBA-2 or RIBA-3) has been replaced by the direct detection of HCV RNA. It can be used, however, to determine false positive antibody testing from past infection. Patients who react to two antigens are more likely to have had a past infection than are those who react to only one antigen. The sensitivity of the RIBA assay is the same as EIA, but the specificity is increased.[10]

The CDC recommends that no further testing be performed in an individual who is EIA negative unless he or she is immunosuppressed. In addition, positive EIA results require confirmatory testing using HCV RNA quantification.[11]

Patients who test positive for the HCV antibody should have measurement of HCV RNA using nucleic acid testing (NAT) to confirm active infection and to quantify viremia if treatment is being considered. The presence of HCV RNA can be detected 1–3 weeks after infection, approximately 1 month before the appearance of total anti-HCV antibodies. The persistence of HCV RNA after 6 months denotes chronic HCV infection.

Multiple assays are available to detect and quantify viral load using a combination of amplification and detection techniques. NATs are classified into qualitative tests (qualitative polymerase chain reaction [PCR], transcription-mediated amplification [TMA]) and quantitative tests (branched-chain DNA [bDNA] amplification, quantitative PCR, and real-time PCR). Regardless of which method is used, HCV RNA IU/mL is the preferred quantitative unit and has been implemented in most commercial assays. Normalization to international units allows for comparable results among the different assays. Historically, qualitative assays to detect HCV RNA were more sensitive than quantitative assays. However, with the availability of real-time PCR, this is no longer the case. Real-time PCR has a lower limit of detection of 10–15 IU/mL and a low false-positive rate. For this reason, real-time PCR has become the method of choice to detect and quantify HCV PCR in clinical practice. Detection of HCV RNA in peripheral blood is used clinically to diagnose chronic HCV infection and to monitor the virologic response to antiviral therapy. A negative NAT result following a positive serologic test result is indicative of a resolved infection. However, low-level viremia can occur during chronic infection, so clinicians should perform a second NAT 6–12 months later to confirm the absence of viremia.[12] In addition, a positive HCV NAT result indicates active infection, regardless of antibody test results.

Routine Laboratory Testing

Measuring the alanine aminotransferase (ALT) level is an inexpensive but relatively insensitive way to measure disease activity in hepatitis C. Studies have demonstrated a weak association between the ALT measurement and the histopathologic findings on liver biopsy.[13,14] Approximately 24–40% of patients with chronic HCV have normal ALT levels. Once a diagnosis of chronic hepatitis C has been made, measurement of liver enzymes offers little additional clinical information regarding viral activity and fibrosis, although an aspartate aminotransferase (AST)-to-ALT ratio greater than 1 can be an indicator of cirrhosis.

Thrombocytopenia is often one of the earliest signs of portal hypertension. A complete blood count should be part of the initial evaluation of a patient with hepatitis C. A complete metabolic panel and a prothrombin time/international normalized ratio (PT/INR) are also standard tests ordered. A low serum albumin and an elevated INR can reflect the presence of cirrhosis with hepatocellular dysfunction.

HCV Core Antigen Detection

An immunoassay to detect and quantify total HCV core protein in serum has been developed.[15] HCV core antigen levels have an excellent correlation with HCV RNA concentrations and can be considered an alternative to measuring the HCV RNA level.[16] Automated testing for antibodies to core protein is less expensive than PCR-based assays. However, core antibody testing has not been adopted in clinical practice because of its relatively low sensitivity, with a lower limit of detection of 20,000 IU/mL.

HCV Genotyping

Hepatitis C is classified into six major genotypes, numbered 1 through 6 with subtypes a–c. The genotypes vary in nucleotide sequence by as much as 30%, and subtypes vary by 20%. Seventy-one percent of hepatitis C cases in the United States are infected with HCV genotype 1, including 90% of African-Americans. Genotype 2 accounts for 13.5% of all reported HCV cases in the United States, and genotype 3 accounts for 5.5% of the total cases.[17] The

HCV genotype can be determined by direct sequencing from subgenomic regions of the virus, such as core/E1 or NS5B. Historically, genotype was a strong predictor of response to pegylated interferon (PEG-IFN) and ribavirin (RBV) and was used to determine duration of treatment.[16-18] The availability of HCV protease inhibitors has led to a paradigm shift. Patients with genotype 1 infection are candidates for therapy with the combination of a protease inhibitor (PI), PEG-IFN, and RBV. The first-generation PIs have a lower barrier to resistance for genotype 1a, resulting in higher sustained response rates for genotype 1b. PEG-IFN and RBV remain the treatment of choice for patients with non–genotype 1 infections, for which the PIs have little or no activity. For these reasons, it is standard to obtain HCV genotyping in any patient who is considering undergoing treatment for hepatitis C.

Liver Biopsy

A liver biopsy is not essential to the diagnosis of chronic hepatitis C, and the role of biopsy is evolving as response rates increase and noninvasive tests for hepatic fibrosis improve. Liver biopsy remains the gold standard to quantify inflammation (grade) and fibrosis (stage), which are important in guiding treatment decisions. Biopsy also is useful in identifying concomitant causes of liver disease, as well as documenting the presence of cirrhosis, which has important prognostic and management implications. For example, patients found to have cirrhosis on liver biopsy should be started on a surveillance protocol for hepatocellular carcinoma. Sampling error does exist, and specimens shorter than 2 cm can be difficult to interpret.

Liver biopsy findings in a patient with chronic hepatitis C usually consist of a portal lymphocytic infiltrate that may extend and involve the limiting plate. The degree of inflammation and fibrosis can predict the likelihood that a patient will progress to more advanced stages of fibrosis.[18] For this reason, the AASLD guidelines recommend consideration of antiviral therapy for patients with stage II fibrosis or greater in an effort to prevent development of cirrhosis. Treatment of naïve genotype 1 patients with lesser degrees of fibrosis or without fibrosis staging will likely become common practice now that PIs provide sustained response rates exceeding 70% for this group.[19,20]

Noninvasive Assessment of Liver Fibrosis

While liver biopsy has been the preferred method to stage hepatitis C, it has several limitations as well as the risks of pain (20%), bleeding, and hemobilia (0.5%).[21] Sampling error and intraobserver variability affect the diagnostic accuracy of liver biopsy, even with the use of widely validated histologic scoring systems. As a result, noninvasive diagnosis of liver fibrosis has evolved rapidly over recent years. Fibrosis can be detected and quantified by assays that measure serum markers and by an imaging technique that detects liver stiffness (transient elastography). The AST-platelet ratio index (APRI) is a validated and widely studied scoring system that is readily available at low cost. It is most effective at excluding significant HCV-related fibrosis.[22] It is defined by the following formula: [{AST (IU/l)/ ALT_ULN (IU/L)} × 100]/ platelet count (10^9/L). An APRI of less than 0.5 suggests that there is no or minimal fibrosis; an APRI above 1.5 is suggestive of more significant fibrosis. Most scoring systems include a combination of routine laboratory tests with serum biomarkers of fibrosis. Some of these scores have been widely validated in large cohorts of patients (FIBROSpect II, FibroTest, HepaScore)[23–26] and are used in clinical practice. The majority of the scoring systems, including the imaging studies, are very accurate in identifying patients with advanced or no fibrosis, but their sensitivity and specificity drop significantly when evaluating for intermediate stages of fibrosis.[27] These measurements of liver fibrosis have not been introduced into the practice guidelines as standard of care, but they do have some value in the assessment of liver fibrosis, especially in patients who are not candidates for liver biopsy or as a means of obtaining serial measurements of fibrosis.

Pharmacogenetics Testing

Recent genome-wide association studies have demonstrated a link between a genetic polymorphism near the *IL28B* gene region and response to PEG-IFN-α plus RBV in patients with genotype 1 chronic HCV.[28–30] These genetic variations have also been found to be associated with spontaneous clearance of the virus without treatment.[31,32] During genetic analysis, the C allele was found to be the strongest established pretreatment predictor of treatment response in HCV genotype 1 patients. Eighty percent of European patients with the C/C genotype cleared the virus, whereas only approximately 30% of those with the T/T genotype did. Interestingly, the favorable genotype was more commonly found in European Americans (39%) compared to African-Americans (16%). This may, in part, explain the well-documented difference in response rates between these two groups of patients. Although initially described in genotype 1 patients, a recent study confirms that the presence of C/C genotype also confers an improved response in genotype 2 and 3 patients.[33]

IL28B genotyping has multiple potential roles for clinical practice. Patients who have the favorable genotype could be selected to undergo treatment with PEG-IFN with sustained virologic response (SVR) rates comparable to the addition of a PI, but with a reduced cost and side-effect profile. In a retrospective analysis of the REALIZE trial, *IL28b* genotyping was no longer a predictor of response. Patients with any of the genotypes had response rates exceeding 60%, suggesting that IL28B genotyping may be of limited utility with the addition of telaprevir.[34] Boceprevir also improved SVR rates in nearly all of the *IL28B* genotype subgroups, with the exception of treatment-naïve patients of the C/C genotype (who exhibited high SVR rates regardless of regimen) and previously treated patients with the T/T genotype who received response-guided boceprevir plus PEG-IFN/RBV.[35]

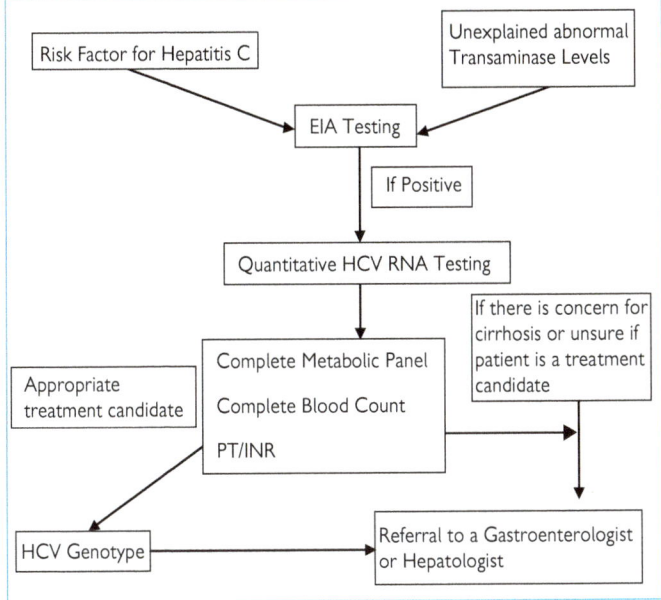

Figure 4.2 Testing algorithm for hepatitis C
Source: © 2011, Natasha Walzer, MD

Conclusion

The decision to screen a patient for hepatitis C should be based on the presence of elevated aminotransferase levels, a risk factor for the acquisition for hepatitis C as stated in the AASLD guidelines, and, in accordance with the proposed CDC recommendations, anyone born between from 1945 and 1965. Screening is performed by EIA testing, and active infection is confirmed by measuring HCV RNA (Figure 4.2). Hepatitis C genotype should be determined in potential treatment candidates. Liver biopsy can be performed to stage the liver disease and to assess for other causes of liver injury. Alternatively, noninvasive assays can provide an indication of the degree of fibrosis. Even if a patient is not thought to be an appropriate candidate for treatment of hepatitis C, documenting the presence of cirrhosis or advanced fibrosis has significant health implications, including a risk of liver failure and hepatocellular carcinoma. Proper screening and evaluation of patients with HCV is critical in bringing affected individuals to medical attention so that they can benefit from recent advances in antiviral therapy.

References

1. Rein DB, Smith BD, Wittenborn JS, et al. The cost-effectiveness of birth-cohort screening for hepatitis C antibody in US primary care settings. *Ann Intern Med.* 2012;156(4):263–270.

2. Alter MJ, Seeff LB, Bacon BR. Testing for hepatitis C virus infection should be routine for persons at increased risk for infection. *Ann Inter Med.* 2004;141:715–717.

3. Beld M, Penning M, van Putten M, et al. Low levels of hepatitis C virus RNA in serum, plasma, and peripheral blood mononuclear cells of injecting drug users during long antibody-undetectable periods before seroconversion. *Blood.* 1999;94:1183–1191.

4. Gretch DR, Wilson JJ, Carithers RL, Jr., et al. Detection of hepatitis C virus RNA: comparison of one-stage polymerase chain reaction (PCR) with nested-set PCR. *J Clin Microbiol.* 1993;31:289–291.

5. Alborino F, Burighel A, Tiller FW, et al. Multicenter evaluation of a fully automated third-generation anti-HCV antibody screening test with excellent sensitivity and specificity. *Med Microbiol Immunol.* 2011;200:77–83.

6. Lok AS, Chien D, Choo QL, et al. Antibody response to core, envelope and nonstructural hepatitis C virus antigens: comparison of immunocompetent and immunosuppressed patients. *Hepatology.* 1993;18:497–502.

7. Pereira BJ, Levey AS. Hepatitis C virus infection in dialysis and renal transplantation. *Kidney Int.* 1997;51:981–999.

8. Pereira BJ, Milford EL, Kirkman RL, et al. Prevalence of hepatitis C virus RNA in organ donors positive for hepatitis C antibody and in the recipients of their organs. *N Engl J Med.* 1992;327:910–915.

9. Lee SR, Kardos KW, Schiff E, et al. Evaluation of a new, rapid test for detecting HCV infection, suitable for use with blood or oral fluid. *J Virol Methods.* 2011;172:27–31.

10. Tobler LH, Lee SR, Stramer SL, et al. Performance of second- and third-generation RIBAs for confirmation of third-generation HCV EIA-reactive blood donations. Retrovirus Epidemiology Donor Study. *Transfusion.* 2000;40:917–923.

11. Alter MJ, Kuhnert WL, Finelli L. Guidelines for laboratory testing and result reporting of antibody to hepatitis C virus. *MMWR.* 2003. http://www.cdc.gov/mmwr/preview/mmwrhtml/rr5203a1.htm

12. Scott JD, McMahon BJ, Bruden D, et al. High rate of spontaneous negativity for hepatitis C virus RNA after establishment of chronic infection in Alaska Natives. *Clin Infect Dis.* 2006;42:945–952.

13. Inglesby TV, Rai R, Astemborski J, et al. A prospective, community-based evaluation of liver enzymes in individuals with hepatitis C after drug use. *Hepatology.* 1999;29:590–596.

14. Marcellin P, Levy S, Erlinger S. Therapy of hepatitis C: patients with normal aminotransferase levels. *Hepatology.* 1997;26:133S–136S.

15. Laperche S, Le Marrec N, Simon N, et al. A new HCV core antigen assay based on disassociation of immune complexes: an alternative to molecular biology in the diagnosis of early HCV infection. *Transfusion.* 2003;43:958–962.

16. Veillon P, Payan C, Picchio G, et al. Comparative evaluation of the total hepatitis C virus core antigen, branched-DNA, and amplicor monitor assays in determining viremia for patients with chronic hepatitis C during interferon plus ribavirin combination therapy. *J Clin Microbiol.* 2003;41:3212–3220.

17. Lau JY, Mizokami M, Kolberg JA, et al. Application of six hepatitis C virus genotyping systems to sera from chronic hepatitis C patients in the United States. *Journal of Infectious Diseases.* 1995;171:281–289.

18. Yano M, Kumada H, Kage M, et al. The long-term pathological evolution of chronic hepatitis C. *Hepatology*. 1996;23:1334–1340.

19. Jacobson IM, McHutchison JG, Dusheiko G, et al. Telaprevir for previously untreated chronic hepatitis C virus infection. *N Engl J Med*. 2011;364:2405–2416.

20. Poordad F, Bronowicki J-P, Gordon SC, et al. *IL28B polymorphism predicts virologic response in patients with hepatitis C genotype 1 treated with boceprevir (BOC) combination therapy*. Program and abstracts of the 46th Annual Meeting of the European Association for the Study of the Liver, March 30–April 3, 2011, Berlin, Germany. Abstract 12.

21. Cadranel JF, Rufat P, & Degos F. Practices of liver biopsy in France: results of a prospective nationwide survey. For the Group of Epidemiology of the French Association for the Study of the Liver (AFEF). *Hepatology*. 2000;32:477–481.

22. Shaheen AA, Myers RP Diagnostic accuracy of the aspartate aminotransferase-to-platelet ratio index for the prediction of hepatitis C-related fibrosis: a systematic review. *Hepatology*. 2007;46:912–921.

23. Adams LA, Bulsara M, Rossi E, et al. Hepascore: an accurate validated predictor of liver fibrosis in chronic hepatitis C infection. *Clin Chem*. 2005; 51:1867–1873.

24. Cales P, Oberti F, Michalak S, et al. A novel panel of blood markers to assess the degree of liver fibrosis. *Hepatology*. 2005;42:1373–1381.

25. Forns X, Ampurdanes S, Llovet JM, et al. Identification of chronic hepatitis C patients without hepatic fibrosis by a simple predictive model. *Hepatology*. 2002;36:986–992.

26. Imbert-Bismut F, Ratziu V, Pieroni L, et al. Biochemical markers of liver fibrosis in patients with hepatitis C virus infection: a prospective study. *Lancet*. 2001;357:1069–1075.

27. Parkes J, Guha IN, Roderick P, Rosenberg W. Performance of serum marker panels for liver fibrosis in chronic hepatitis C. *J Hepatology*. 2006;44:462–474.

28. Ge D, Fellay J, Thompson AJ, et al. Genetic variation in IL28B predicts hepatitis C treatment-induced viral clearance. *Nature*. 2009;461:399–401.

29. Suppiah V, Moldovan M, Ahlenstiel G, et al. IL28B is associated with response to chronic hepatitis C interferon-alpha and ribavirin therapy. *Nat Genet*. 2009;41:1100–1104.

30. Tanaka Y, Nishida N, Sugiyama M, et al. Genome-wide association of IL28B with response to pegylated interferon-alpha and ribavirin therapy for chronic hepatitis C. *Nat Genet*. 2009;41:1105–1109.

31. Rauch A, Kutalik Z, Descombes P, et al. Genetic variation in IL28B is associated with chronic hepatitis C and treatment failure: a genome-wide association study. *Gastroenterology* 2010;138:1338–1345.

32. Thomas DL, Thio CL, Martin MP, et al. Genetic variation in IL28B and spontaneous clearance of hepatitis C virus. *Nature*. 2009;461:798–801.

33. Mangia A, Thompson AJ, Santoro R, et al. An IL28B polymorphism determines treatment response of hepatitis C virus genotype 2 or 3 patients who do not achieve a rapid virologic response. *Gastroenterology*. 2010;139:821–827.

34. Pol S, Aerssens J, Zeuzem S, et al. *Similar SVR rates in IL28B CC, CT or TT prior relapser, partial- or null-responder patients treated with telaprevir/peginter-feron/ribavirin: retrospective analysis of the REALIZE study*. Program and abstracts of the 46th Annual Meeting of the European Association for the Study of the Liver, March 30–April 3, 2011, Berlin, Germany. Abstract 13.

35. Poordad F, McCone J, Jr., Bacon BR, et al. Boceprevir for untreated chronic HCV genotype 1 infection. *N Engl J Med*. 2011;364:1195–1206.

Centers for Disease Control and Prevention (CDC). *Recommendations for Chronic HCV Infection.* http://www.cdc.gov/hepatitis/HCV/GuidelinesC.htm. Updated March 20, 2012. Accessed June 13, 2012.

Chapter 5

Pathology of Viral Hepatitis C

Shriram Jakate

Hepatitis C virus (HCV), an enveloped single-stranded RNA virus classified in the genus *Hepacivirus* in the *Flaviviridae* family, is a common worldwide infection affecting nearly 3% of the world's population.[1] The infection is transmitted parenterally, and the majority of patients (75–85%) who acquire HCV develop chronic hepatitis. About 20% of patients with chronic HCV hepatitis develop cirrhosis over a period of 20–30 years. In cirrhotic patients, there is a 1–4% annual risk of development of hepatocellular carcinoma (HCC).[2] HCV hepatitis and cirrhosis is the leading indication for orthotopic liver transplantation (OLT) in the United States. However, with the recent advent of direct-acting antivirals (DAAs), these statistics will likely significantly improve in the future. Eradication of virus in the form of undetectable serum HCV RNA (sustained viral response [SVR]) is being achieved with the use of DAAs in the majority of patients. These new therapies result in a decreased rate of chronicity, regression of cirrhosis, a significantly improved clinical outcome and survival, and decreased incidence of complications including HCC.

HCV infection is diagnosed in two steps[3]: (1) serological screening test for anti-HCV antibodies (this does not differentiate between acute or chronic or past and current infection). If this test is positive: (2) a nucleic acid test for HCV RNA for quantitative HCV (viral load) as well as HCV viral genotyping (some of the six genotypes are easier to treat than others[4]). Although the diagnosis of HCV is made serologically, pathological evaluation of the liver tissue is crucial in the management of patients with HCV infection.[5] However, the frequency of liver biopsy for HCV is declining as therapeutic outcomes have advanced and noninvasive methods for detection of fibrosis are becoming available.

The following are the various clinical scenarios where pathological evaluation plays an important role:

1. Acute HCV viral hepatitis (exclusion of potential nonviral causes of acute liver injury)
2. Chronic HCV viral hepatitis, initial pathological assessment (grading of inflammatory activity and staging of fibrosis)
3. Chronic HCV viral hepatitis, follow-up pathological assessment (monitoring of posttherapeutic or nontherapeutic alteration/progression in grade and stage compared with the initial biopsy)

4. HCV coinfection with other viruses (HBV, HIV)
5. HCV coexistent with other chronic liver diseases (such as nonalcoholic fatty liver disease [NAFLD], alcoholic or EtOH hepatitis, and autoimmune hepatitis [AIH])
6. Explanted HCV cirrhotic liver (for dominant nodules including macroregenerative nodules, dysplastic nodules, and HCC)
7. Recurrent HCV hepatitis in the OLT graft (recurrent HCV hepatitis vs. acute cellular rejection [ACR], residual hepatitis after HCV eradication or SVR, and fibrosing cholestatic hepatitis—a rare variant of recurrent HCV hepatitis)

Acute HCV Hepatitis

The term *acute viral hepatitis* is used when hepatic inflammation and elevated serum transaminases levels are present for approximately less than 6 months or 26 weeks.[6] Acute HCV hepatitis is sporadic after parenteral exposure, often clinically undetected in the large majority of patients, and spontaneously resolves in 15–25% of patients.[7] The remainder progress to chronic HCV hepatitis. Liver biopsy is rarely performed in acute HCV hepatitis since the symptoms are either absent or mild and nonspecific. If a liver biopsy is indeed performed during acute HCV hepatitis, it may be primarily to determine if other conditions such as autoimmune hepatitis or steatohepatitis are contributing to the abnormal liver function tests (LFT) pattern. The histological changes of acute HCV hepatitis are nonspecific, but the inflammatory changes are predominantly and disproportionately within the hepatic lobules rather than at the portal–lobular interfaces (the opposite generally occurs in chronic HCV hepatitis). Individual hepatocytes show focal ballooning degeneration ("spotty hepatitis"), which provokes a collection of small clusters of mononuclear inflammatory cells (lymphocytes and macrophages) producing necroinflammatory activity (Figure 5.1). Concomitantly, hepatocytes may display apoptosis with dense eosinophilic cytoplasm and pyknotic nuclei ("acidophil or Councilman bodies") with little or no inflammatory activity (Figure 5.2). These inflammatory lobular changes are common to both acute and chronic viral hepatitis, multiple different viral hepatitis agents, and even other liver diseases. What distinguishes acute from chronic HCV hepatitis is the lack of fibrosis and relative lack of interface chronic inflammatory activity. Occasionally, when acute HCV hepatitis is more severe, there may be additional features such as hepatocellular cholestasis and reactive biliary cholangiolar inflammatory and proliferative changes. None of these histological features is predictive of predisposition or propensity for future chronicity or disease progression.

The most severe form of acute hepatitis is fulminant hepatic necrosis (FHN) or acute hepatic failure (AHF), where there is a rapid decrease in liver synthesis and onset of hepatic encephalopathy within a few weeks. This

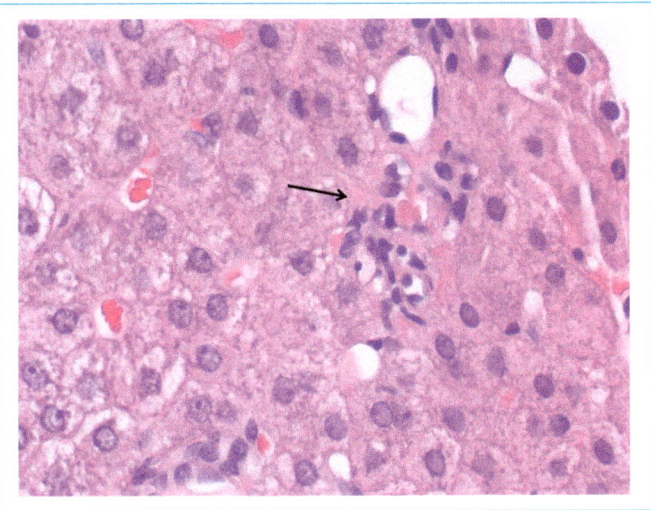

Figure 5.1 High-magnification microphotograph of a hepatic lobule showing focal necrosis of a few hepatocytes (*arrow*) evoking a localized chronic inflammatory cell reaction. This HCV-associated histological finding is also known as spotty hepatitis (H&E stain, ×600 magnification)

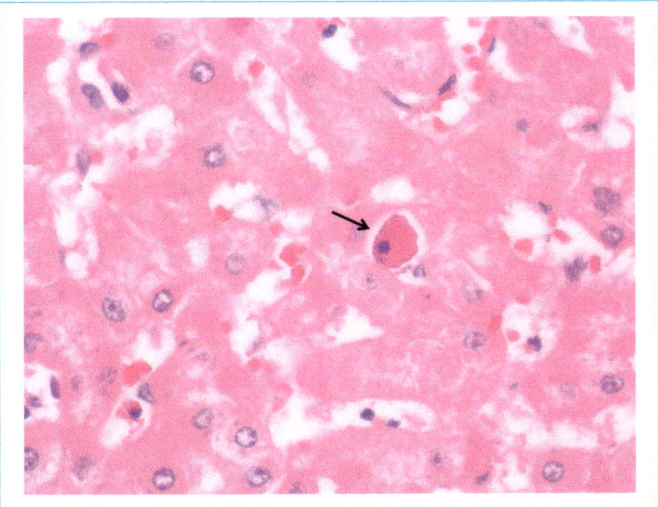

Figure 5.2 High-magnification microphotograph of a hepatic lobule showing an isolated hepatocyte undergoing apoptosis (*arrow*) with densely acidophilic or eosinophilic cytoplasm and a shrunken pyknotic nucleus (acidophil or Councilman body). There are no associated inflammatory cells (H&E stain, ×600 magnification)

is associated with high mortality without liver transplantation. While HCV hepatitis is documented as causing AHF (<1% of HCV cases) in Asia, it is an extremely rare cause for AHF in the United States, where most cases of AHF result from acetaminophen toxicity, idiosyncratic drug reactions, or unknown causes. Histologically, in AHF, instead of necrosis of individual hepatocytes, there is massive hepatocytic destruction with collapse of large segments of hepatic parenchyma. The surviving hepatocytes may regenerate briskly, causing patchy nodularity (an erroneous mimicry to cirrhosis, pathologically). A zonal pattern of necrosis (zones 3 and 2) and eosinophilic degeneration of hepatocytes may histologically distinguish acetaminophen toxicity from other causes of AHF.

Chronic HCV Hepatitis, Initial Pathological Assessment

Chronic HCV hepatitis implies the presence of elevated serum transaminases or hepatic inflammation for more than 6 months. Once the HCV infection becomes chronic, spontaneous resolution of HCV hepatitis is unlikely. The natural history of chronic HCV hepatitis is variable and influenced by multiple host factors (such as other coexistent liver diseases) and viral factors (such as viral load, genotype,[4] and other viral coinfections). Nevertheless, without effective therapy, there is a gradual progression of the disease, with about 20% of patients progressing to cirrhosis over a period of 20–30 years. Pretherapeutic pathological evaluation of chronic HCV hepatitis is important in assessing the baseline level of severity of inflammation (grade) and the extent of disease progression in the form of fibrosis (stage). The histological inflammatory changes in chronic HCV hepatitis are not diagnostic or pathognomonic, but they are generally consistent and diffuse throughout the liver. There are portal discrete aggregates of mature lymphocytes that are preferentially located around or adjacent to the interlobular bile ducts (*periductal or paraductal lymphoid aggregates*, Figure 5.3). These lymphoid aggregates may also have germinal centers. Apart from such discrete lymphoid aggregates, there are increased chronic inflammatory cells (predominantly lymphocytes and macrophages) located within the portal tracts, with variable destruction and encroachment of the lobular limiting plates or portal–lobular interfaces (*interface hepatitis*, previously called *piecemeal necrosis*, Figure 5.4). The inflammatory cells may include a few plasma cells or eosinophils. However, if either of these cell types predominates, conditions such as autoimmune hepatitis and drug-induced liver disease may be coexistent with chronic HCV hepatitis. The extent of interface hepatitis is the most crucial component of chronic HCV grading. The lobular changes of spotty hepatitis and acidophil bodies may also be present, but these are less predominant than portal or periportal inflammation in chronic HCV hepatitis (vs. acute HCV hepatitis). Macrovesicular steatosis is often present in chronic HCV hepatitis,

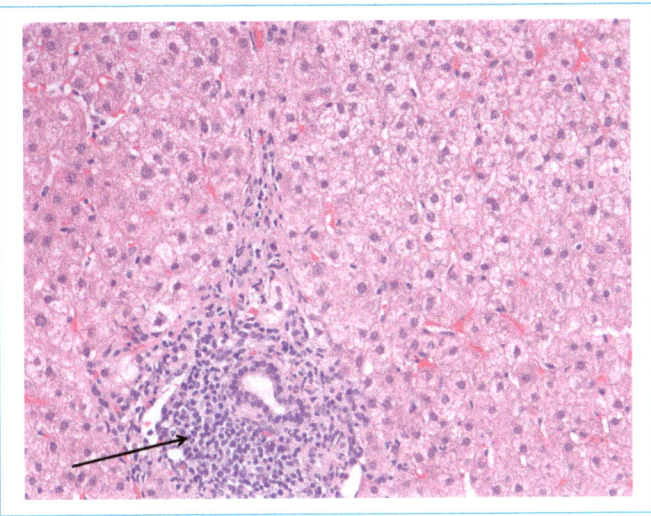

Figure 5.3 Microphotograph of chronic hepatitis C showing a typical paraductal lymphoid aggregate (*arrow*) within the portal tract adjacent to a bile duct (H&E stain, ×200 magnification)

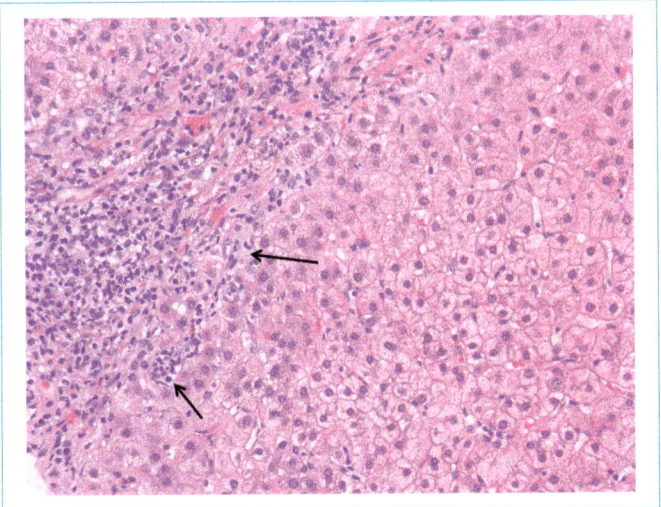

Figure 5.4 Medium-magnification microphotograph showing chronic inflammatory cells patchily involving the portal–lobular interface (*arrows*). This is interface hepatitis or piecemeal necrosis (grade 2/4 chronic HCV hepatitis, H&E stain, ×200 magnification)

but it is focal and seen in a few hepatocytes. However, in HCV genotype 3, moderate to severe hepatic steatosis may be seen.[4] The ongoing portal and periportal inflammation eventually results in fibrosis, which originates in the portal tracts and subsequently involves periportal areas, creates portal–portal and portal–central fibrous bridges (Figure 5.5), and leads to diffuse curvilinear fibrosis and cirrhotic nodularity. In a biopsy sample, it is important to evaluate the degree of fibrosis (staging) in the peripheral smaller portal tracts (recognized by a single portal triad and regular-sized portal vein, hepatic artery, and interlobular bile duct) rather than the larger segmental portal areas (recognized by large-caliber blood vessels and multiple larger bile ducts) which may be misinterpreted as showing a greater than actual stage of fibrosis.

Any of the multiple available grading and staging scoring systems may be utilized to objectively or semi-quantitatively evaluate chronic HCV hepatitis. This is crucial for the baseline assessment as well as for comparing the alterations in the subsequent posttherapeutic or nontherapeutic samples. However, it is important to employ a practical scoring system that is consistently and reproducibly applied, easy to follow, and utilized by the treating hepatologist for patient care. There are various grading and staging scoring systems available (originally by Knodell[8,9] and later modified by Ishak,[10] Batts and Ludwig,[11] Scheuer,[12] and METAVIR[13] or the French Cooperative Study Group). The most frequently used system by practicing pathologists in the United States is Batts and Ludwig (Table 5.1).

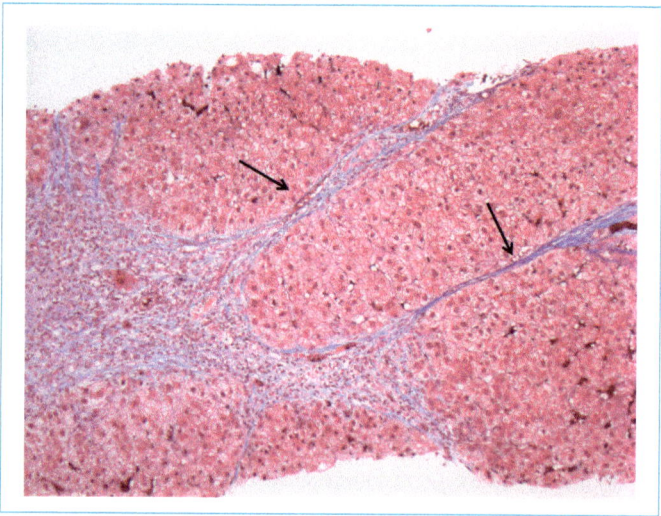

Figure 5.5 Medium-magnification microphotograph showing thin portal-to-portal fibrous strands (*arrows*). The tissue is stained by trichrome stain to highlight the fibrosis. This would be bridging fibrosis or stage 3/4 fibrosis in the staging system for chronic HCV hepatitis (×100 magnification)

Table 5.1 Scoring system for grading and staging

Scoring System for Grading (after Batts and Ludwig)

	Portal/Periportal Inflammation	Lobular Inflammation
Grade 0	None or minimal	None
Grade 1	Portal inflammation only	Inflammatory cells but no hepatocellular death
Grade 2	Mild interface hepatitis	Focal cell death
Grade 3	Moderate interface hepatitis	Severe focal cell death
Grade 4	Severe interface hepatitis	Hepatocellular damage includes bridging necrosis

Scoring System for Staging (after Batts and Ludwig)

Stage 0	No fibrosis
Stage 1	Enlarged fibrotic portal tracts
Stage 2	Periportal fibrous septae, rare portal-portal fibrous septae
Stage 3	Bridging fibrosis with architectural distortion but no obvious cirrhosis
Stage 4	Probable or definite cirrhosis

Chronic HCV Hepatitis, Follow-up Pathological Assessment

Follow-up pathological evaluation of chronic HCV hepatitis may be required in multiple clinical settings such as untreated HCV with potentially worsening disease, treated HCV with limited or no clinical improvement, and treated HCV with clinical improvement. The pathological changes are expected to generally correlate with these clinical conditions. For the sake of accuracy, it may be helpful to simultaneously review the original as well as the follow-up samples for grading and staging and employ a practical and consistent scoring system. Two factors that will likely influence this follow-up pathological assessment in the near future include increasing use of noninvasive fibrosis assessment methods (such as ultrasonic transient elastography) and the effectiveness of DAAs. For now, liver biopsy is still a generally preferred method of fibrosis assessment compared to the noninvasive methods. And the extent and rate of resolution of hepatitis and fibrosis after virological cure (SVR) currently remains indeterminate.[14] Untreated HCV during follow-up usually shows worsening of grade and stage over long periods of time. Conversely, successfully treated HCV shows variable but significant resolution in both grade and stage. Even fibrosis that was earlier regarded as irreversible is known to show regression after SVR.[15]

HCV Coinfection with Other Viruses

HCV and HBV

Both hepatitis C and hepatitis B viruses are major global public health problems. Dual infection by HCV and HBV may occur due to their shared modes of transmission and high prevalence in endemic areas and high-risk populations.[16,17] Approximately 10–15% of patients with chronic HBV infection are also infected with HCV. Rather than simultaneous infection, the most common sequence is HCV superinfection in previously HBV-infected patients. Patients with dual viral hepatitis infections carry a greater risk of advanced liver disease, cirrhosis, and HCC compared with monoinfected patients. Additionally, successful therapy for one of the two viruses may result in reactivation of the other virus. Histologically, along with the usual pattern of chronic hepatitis C (portal lymphoid aggregates, interface hepatitis, and lobular spotty hepatitis), features typical for chronic HBV hepatitis may also be present. These include hepatocellular cytoplasmic ground-glass change (usually immunohistochemically positivity for HBsAg) and hepatocellular nuclear finely granular inclusions or "sanded nuclei" (usually immunohistochemically positivity for HBcAg). The grading and scoring system employed for dual infections is the same as in monoinfection.

HCV and HIV

Overall, up to 10% of patients with HIV have HCV coinfection in the Western population.[18] However, the prevalence of HCV in HIV is highest among injection drug users (>50%). HIV has a negative impact on natural progression of HCV, including persistence of high viral load and more rapid progression to cirrhosis and hepatic decompensation. Histologically, the HIV-HCV coinfected patients show primarily chronic HCV hepatitis-related changes. Potential additional histologic changes may include drug hepatotoxicity, steatosis, and steatohepatitis.

HCV Coexistent with other Chronic Liver Diseases

Multiple chronic liver diseases such as EtOH hepatitis, NAFLD, and autoimmune hepatitis are fairly common in the population. Hence, coexistence of one or more of these diseases along with HCV hepatitis can be clinically anticipated. Histologically, it may pose challenges in terms of assessing the burden or dominance of one disease process versus the other, particularly for therapeutic precedence.

HCV and AIH

Both chronic HCV and AIH can histologically mimic each other since interface chronic inflammatory activity is common in both. Their separate histological recognition is important given the potentially variable disease progressions and divergent and conflicting therapeutic choices. Apart from the usual histologic changes of chronic HCV hepatitis, in cases of coexistent AIH, there are prominent interface plasma cells and rosettes and noticeable mature lymphocytes in the sinusoidal spaces. Even with these compelling histological features, serological correlation (elevated autoantibodies and gamma globulins) is needed for confirming the coexistence of both diseases.

HCV and NAFLD

HCV is known to be associated with metabolic alterations that may result in steatosis, insulin resistance, metabolic syndrome, and diabetes.[19,20] Both HCV and NAFDL may also coexist, given their frequency in the population, and each may adversely influence the severity of the other. A few hepatocytes showing incidental macrovesicular steatosis is common in all genotypes of HCV. However, HCV genotype 3 is typically associated with moderate to severe steatosis.[4] Coexistent NAFLD related to host factors may be suspected when the macrovesicular steatosis is associated with ballooning, steatohepatitis, and increased hepatocellular nuclear and cytoplasmic glycogen.

HCV and EtOH Hepatitis

EtOH hepatitis adversely affects HCV hepatitis since it has a synergistic effect on oxidative stress, immune reaction, and carcinogenesis.[21] This causes significant increase in the risk for cirrhosis and HCC. Apart from HCV-related findings, there may be prominent macrovesicular steatosis, ballooning, Mallory bodies, neutrophilic inflammatory response, and perivenular fibrosis suggestive of EtOH.

Explanted HCV Cirrhotic Liver

Decompensated HCV-related cirrhosis with or without HCC is the most common indication for liver transplantation in Western countries. Although the rate of fibrosis in chronic HCV hepatitis is variable, about 20–30% of patients eventually progress to cirrhosis and are at risk of hepatic decompensation. With HCV-related cirrhosis, both direct and indirect pathways of carcinogenesis are responsible for HCC development (1–4% annual risk). The explanted cirrhotic liver typically shows variably sized cirrhotic nodules ("mixed nodular cirrhosis," Figure 5.6) and microscopically usual features of HCV hepatitis.

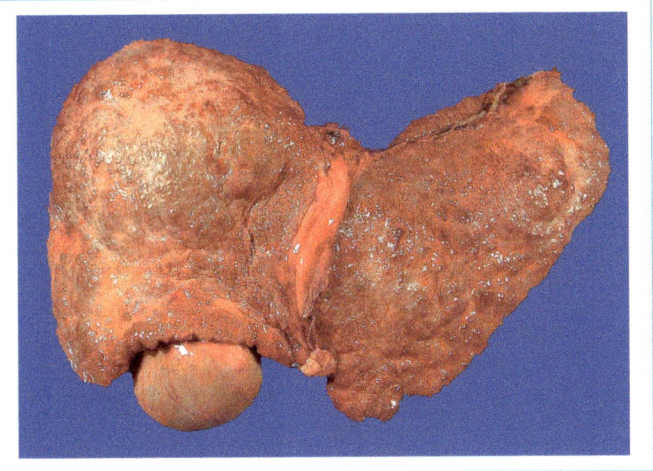

Figure 5.6 Explanted liver with HCV cirrhosis (external and anterior aspect) showing postnecrotic mixed nodularity with bosselated external surface

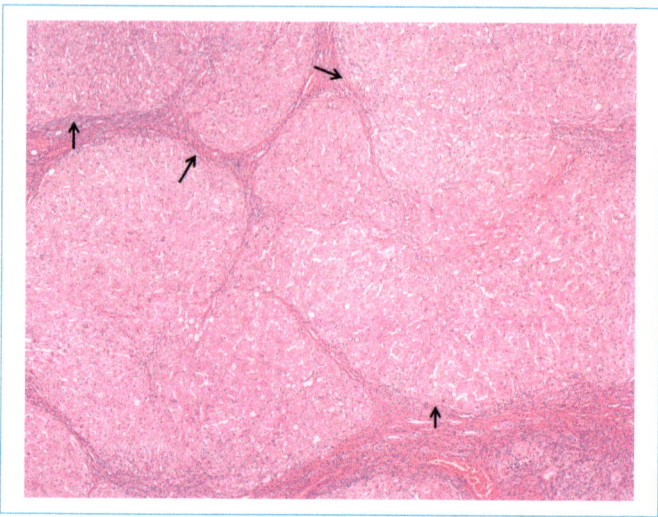

Figure 5.7 Low-magnification microphotograph from the explanted liver showing cirrhotic nodularity (stage 4/4 fibrosis) and relatively diminished inflammatory activity (*arrows*) around the portal-lobular interfaces (H&E stain, ×40 magnification)

The extent of inflammatory activity (grade) may or may not be necessarily concordant with the highest stage of fibrosis (stage 4 fibrosis or cirrhosis). Often, the inflammatory activity is diminished in advanced fibrosis (Figure 5.7). HCC nodule(s) detected clinically (on imaging) are identified and examined microscopically to determine the grade and stage of HCC. Previously treated HCC nodules (i.e., chemoembolization or radioembolization) are examined for the degree of therapeutic necrosis and potential residual viable tumor. Additionally, clinically undetected but grossly abnormal appearing nodules are evaluated to determine if these are benign macroregenerative nodules, nodules with dysplasia, or previously undetected nodules of HCC.

Recurrent HCV Hepatitis in the OLT Graft

Unfortunately, HCV is not eliminated by transplantation, and reinfection of the graft occurs universally at reperfusion.[22,23] However, severity of recurrent disease, level of graft dysfunction, and rate of fibrosis progression are extremely variable. Overall, post-OLT HCV recurrence shows higher viremia and faster fibrosis progression (20–30% develop cirrhosis within 5 years after OLT[24]). The early recurrent HCV hepatitis is identified by HCV RNA levels clinically but may be somewhat challenging to histologically differentiate from ACR. Recurrent HCV hepatitis shows essentially similar inflammatory changes as in the native liver (lobular spotty hepatitis, apoptotic bodies, portal focal lymphoid aggregates, and interface inflammatory activity). This needs to be differentiated from ACR, which shows diffuse and dense portal

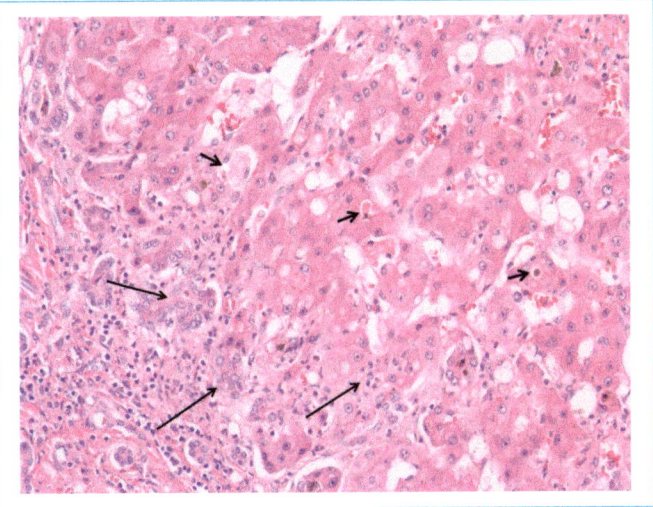

Figure 5.8 Medium-magnification microphotograph showing histological features of fibrosing cholestatic hepatitis: lobular cholestasis with hepatocellular canalicular bile and feathery degeneration (*short arrows*) and reactive cholangiolar proliferation and acute cholangiolitis (*long arrows*, H&E stain, ×200 magnification)

infiltrates that include mature and reactive lymphoid cells, eosinophils, and macrophages in addition to selective inflammatory targeting of portal and hepatic veins ("endotheliitis") and bile ducts ("ductulitis"). With more effective HCV therapies, a newly emerging histological entity is residual and ongoing hepatitis, apparently histologically suggestive of recurrent HCV hepatitis but with clinical SVR. Whether or not this has similar risk of fibrosis progression is yet to be defined.

An uncommon form of aggressive HCV recurrence (<10%) is fibrosing cholestatic hepatitis (FCH).[22] Clinically, this is defined by very high serum HCV RNA levels, high bilirubin and alkaline phosphatase levels, absence of biliary obstruction or surgical biliary complications, absence of hepatic artery thrombosis, and relatively early period of posttransplantation (1–6 months).[23] Histologically, cholestatic features dominate with hepatocytes showing canalicular cholestasis and ballooning degeneration along with cholangiolar or bile ductular proliferation, cholangiolitis, and periportal fibrosis (Figure 5.8). The histological features are not specific, but FCH may be suspected when there is clinically high viremia and absence of obstructive, vascular, or toxic injury.

References

1. Khachatoorian R, French SW. Chaperones in hepatitis C virus infection. *World J Hepatol*. 2016;8(1):9–35.

2. Tholey DM, Ahn J. Impact of hepatitis C virus infection on hepatocellular carcinoma. *Gastroenterol Clin North Am*. 2015;44(4):761–773.

3. Cloherty G, Talal A, Coller K, et al. Role of serologic and molecular diagnostic assays in identification and management of hepatitis C virus infection. *J Clin Microbiol*. 2016;54(2):265–273.

4. Chan A, Patel K, Naggie S. Genotype 3 infection: the last stand of hepatitis C virus. *Drugs*. 2017;77(2):131–144.

5. Dhingra S, Ward SC, Thung SN. Liver pathology of hepatitis C, beyond grading and staging of the disease. *World J Gastroenterol*. 2016;22(4):1357–1366.

6. Martinello M, Matthews GV. Enhancing the detection and management of acute hepatitis C virus infection. *Int J Drug Policy*. 2015;26(10):899–910.

7. Lingala S, Ghany MG. Natural history of hepatitis C. *Gastroenterol Clin North Am*. 2015;44(4):717–734.

8. Knodell RG, Ishak KG, Black WC, et al. Formulation and application of a numerical scoring system for assessing histological activity in asymptomatic chronic active hepatitis. *Hepatology*. 1981;1(5):431–435.

9. Desmet VJ, Knodell RG, Ishak KG, Black WC, Chen TS, Craig R, Kaplowitz N, Kiernan TW, Wollman J. Formulation and application of a numerical scoring system for assessing histological activity in asymptomatic chronic active hepatitis [hepatology 1981;1:431–435]. *J Hepatol*. 2003;38(4):382–386.

10. Ishak K, Baptista A, Bianchi L, et al. Histological grading and staging of chronic hepatitis. *J Hepatol*. 1995;22(6):696–699.

11. Batts KP, Ludwig J. Chronic hepatitis: an update on terminology and reporting. *Am J Surg Pathol*. 1995;19(12):1409–1417.

12. Scheuer PJ. Classification of chronic viral hepatitis: a need for reassessment. *J Hepatol*. 1991;13(3):372–374.

13. Bedossa P, Poynard T. An algorithm for the grading of activity in chronic hepatitis C. The METAVIR cooperative study group. *Hepatology*. 1996;24(2):289–293.

14. D'Ambrosio R, Degasperi E, Aghemo A, et al. Serological tests do not predict residual fibrosis in hepatitis C cirrhotics with a sustained virological response to interferon. *PLoS One*. 2016;11(6):e0155967.

15. Lee YA, Friedman SL. Reversal, maintenance or progression: what happens to the liver after a virologic cure of hepatitis C? *Antiviral Res*. 2014;107:23–30.

16. Bojito-Marrero L, Pyrsopoulos N. Hepatitis B and hepatitis C reactivation in the biologic era. *J Clin Transl Hepatol*. 2014;2(4):240–246.

17. Konstantinou D, Deutsch M. The spectrum of HBV/HCV coinfection: epidemiology, clinical characteristics, viral interactions and management. *Ann Gastroenterol*. 2015;28(2):221–228.

18. Tsochatzis EA, Castera L. Assessing liver disease in HIV-HCV coinfected patients. *Curr Opin HIV AIDS*. 2015;10(5):316–322.

19. Gastaldi G, Goossens N, Clement S, Negro F. Current level of evidence on causal association between hepatitis C virus and type 2 diabetes: a review. *J Adv Res*. 2017;8(2):149–159.

20. Chang ML. Metabolic alterations and hepatitis C: from bench to bedside. *World J Gastroenterol*. 2016;22(4):1461–1476.

21. Testino G, Leone S, Borro P. Alcoholic liver disease and the hepatitis C virus: an overview and a point of view. *Minerva Med*. 2016;107(5):300–313.

22. Hori T, Onishi Y, Kamei H, et al. Fibrosing cholestatic hepatitis C in post-transplant adult recipients of liver transplantation. *Ann Gastroenterol*. 2016;29(4):454–459.

23. Rubin A, Aguilera V, Berenguer M. Liver transplantation and hepatitis C. *Clin Res Hepatol Gastroenterol*. 2011;35(12):805–812.
24. Felmlee DJ, Coilly A, Chung RT, Samuel D, Baumert TF. New perspectives for preventing hepatitis C virus liver graft infection. *Lancet Infect Dis*. 2016;16(6):735–745.

Chapter 6

Acute Hepatitis C

Christin N. Price and Arthur Y. Kim

The majority of hepatitis C virus (HCV) infections in the United States occurred during the 1970s and 1980s (see Chapter 2), but, in the past decade, a new epidemic of HCV is occurring primarily related to a resurgence of injection drug use. In addition to people who inject drugs (PWID), another increasingly recognized group at risk for acute HCV includes men who have sex with men (MSM), particularly those with preexisting HIV infection. Since the vast majority of infections are asymptomatic, detecting an early-stage HCV infection is a clinical challenge. The identification of acute HCV requires knowledge of behavioral risk factors and proper interpretation of diagnostic tests. It is especially important to identify acute HCV because earlier identification allows for preventive interventions, and treatment of acute HCV infection may interrupt further transmission.

Definition

While definitions vary in the literature, acute hepatitis C infection can be defined as the first 6 months after infection. It is during this period when spontaneous clearance of virus may occur, and the efficacy of early antiviral treatments is maximal. Figure 6.1 displays the natural history of acute HCV for both those who spontaneously clear infection (Figure 6.1A) and those who develop persistent or chronic infection (Figure 6.1B).

Incidence

After the implementation of blood product screening for HCV infection and a decrease in rates of injection drug use, the incidence of acute hepatitis C infection declined after reaching a peak in 1992. This decline in acute infections continued until 2005, when the levels reached a plateau.[1] In 2014, a total of 2,194 cases of acute hepatitis C were reported to US Centers for Disease Control (CDC) from 40 states. The overall incidence rate for 2014 was 0.7 cases per 100,000 population, an increase from 2010–2012. After adjusting for underascertainment and underreporting, an estimated 30,500 acute hepatitis C cases occurred in 2014. In 2014, among all age groups, persons aged 20–29 years had the highest rate (2.20 cases per 100,000 population) of acute HCV infection.

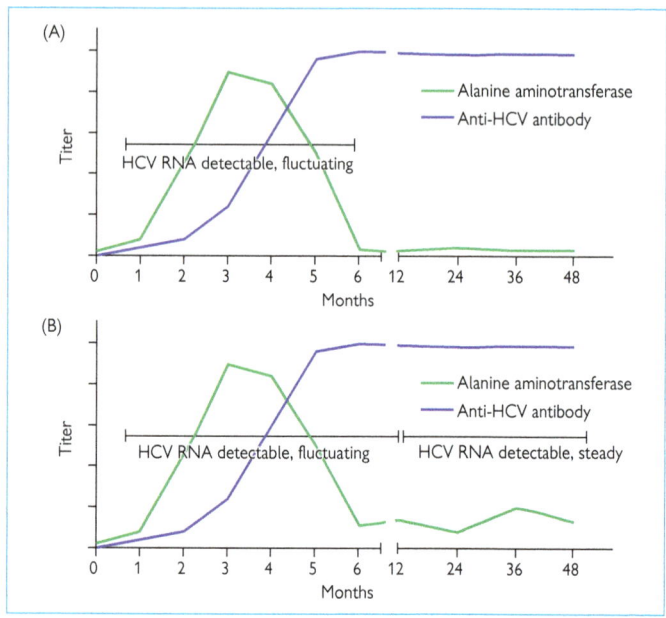

Figure 6.1 Outcomes of acute HCV. (A) Course of HCV infection and spontaneous resolution. (B) Course of HCV infection and progression to chronic infection. Key points include the appearance of HCV RNA prior to ALT elevation and development of antibody and that the acute infection period includes HCV RNA fluctuations that often exceed 1 log

More recently, there has been a concerning rise in rates of acute HCV infection among young individuals in certain regions of the United States. State surveillance reports from 2006 to 2012 reveal the largest increases in reported cases of acute HCV infection occurring east of the Mississippi River, particularly among states in central Appalachia.[2] The majority of these cases occurred in individuals younger than 30 years, with 73% citing injection drug use (IDU) as the principal risk factor. In Massachusetts, rates of confirmed acute HCV infection rose from 1.4 per 100,000 population in 2007 to 3.9 per 100,000 in 2014.[3] Of the acute HCV cases that occurred during this time period (n = 1596), 60.4% were associated with IDU. Historically, acute HCV infection rates have been higher among males in all age groups. However, in 2008, the CDC reported for the first time that acute HCV infection rates were equal (0.3 cases per 100,000 population) between males and females. In 2014, rates among males and females were 0.8 and 0.7 cases per 100,000 population, respectively.

With respect to race and ethnicity, acute HCV infection rates had been highest among American Indian/Alaskan Natives and Blacks, with lower rates occurring among Caucasians and Hispanics during the initial epidemic in the 1970s and 1980s. However, while incidence rates have increased among all racial/ethnic groups since 2002, there has been a shift in IDU behaviors by ethnicity.[4] By 2014, rates of acute hepatitis C among American Indians/Alaska Natives were highest (1.32 per 100,000 population) followed by White non-Hispanics (0.84 per 100,000 population). Black non-Hispanics were significantly lower, with an incidence rate of 0.25 per 100,000 population.

There has also been a reported increase in sexually acquired acute HCV infection among MSM, with especially higher rates seen in HIV-infected MSM.[5]

Other potential routes of transmission leading to acute HCV include nosocomial (exposure to contaminated needles/syringes/multiuse vials), occupational (e.g., needlestick), unsafe tattoos, and intranasal cocaine. Household transmission is extremely rare and may involve sharing of razors or toothbrushes (see Chapter 2).

Clinical Features

The majority of acute HCV infections are asymptomatic, and clinically apparent jaundice is often absent. Of the 20–30% of patients who become symptomatic with acute HCV infection, the most common symptoms are nonspecific and include fatigue, myalgias, right upper quadrant abdominal pain, nausea/vomiting, and poor appetite. Only 10–20% of patients experience clinical evidence of hepatitis (elevated alanine aminotransferase >10 times the upper limit of normal) and jaundice.[6] In the minority of cases that are symptomatic, acute hepatitis occurs 2–12 weeks after the exposure and can last an additional 2–12 weeks. Acute infection progresses to fulminant liver failure on extremely rare occasion. Extrahepatic manifestations of chronic hepatitis C infection, such as vasculitis, cryoglobulinemia, porphyria cutanea tarda, and membranous glomerulonephritis are not associated with acute infection.

During this period, individuals may spontaneously clear the virus on their own (approximately 20% of those infected). Jaundice at presentation, female gender, younger age at acquisition, and non–African-American race are associated with spontaneous clearance.[7] However, the remaining 80% go on to develop chronic HCV infection, and, of these, up to 20% will go on to develop cirrhosis and other complications of liver disease (see Chapter 3).

Diagnosis

The diagnosis of acute HCV infection is a clinical one based on risk factors, known exposures, and symptoms followed by confirmatory testing. This is summarized in Box 6.1.

History

The fact that 85–90% of cases of acute hepatitis C infection are asymptomatic makes an assessment by history for behavioral risk factors crucial to identify acute HCV infection. High-risk groups are listed in Box 6.2. The most common risk factor for acquiring acute HCV remains IDU. The incidence of HCV infection is between 20 and 40 infections per 100 person-years in those who inject drugs. The timing of *initiation* of injecting drugs is also crucial to determining

> **Box 6.1 Diagnosis of Acute HCV**
>
> **Definite**
>
> Seroconversion (positive anti-HCV antibody with negative HCV in the past year)
>
> Seronegative window (HCV RNA positive with negative anti-HCV antibody, subsequent seroconversion)
>
> **Probable**
>
> History of recent high-risk exposures and/or recent illness consistent with acute HCV
>
> **Supporting Data**
>
> Elevated LFTs in absence of other causes
> HCV antibody-positive
> HCV RNA fluctuations >1.0 log
> HCV RNA <10^5 IU/mL
> Spontaneous clearance of HCV

an individual's risk for acquiring new HCV infection; the highest rates are among individuals who just started injecting drugs within the past 12 months.[8] Likewise, a detailed history of *habits* while using IV drugs is also important, as rates of sharing syringes have declined in developed countries, yet sharing drug paraphernalia (e.g., cookers, cottons) is still relatively common and has

> **Box 6.2 High Risk Groups and Historical Features that Should Increase Suspicion for Acute HCV**
>
> **Injection drug users**
>
> Initiation of IDU in past year
>
> New behaviors (sharing equipment, including syringes, cookers, filtration cotton, rinse water)
>
> New partners with whom drug paraphernalia is shared
>
> Previously tested negative for HCV infection
>
> Elevated liver function tests
>
> Men who have sex with men, HIV+
>
> **Practices resulting in semen-to-blood or blood-to-blood exposure:**
> - Receptive anal intercourse (unprotected) with visible blood
> - Fisting
> - Sex toys
>
> Group sex
>
> Sex under the influence of drugs
>
> Elevated liver function tests

been associated with a threefold higher rate of seroconversion compared with those who share no paraphernalia.[9] Among non-IDU, there is little evidence that exists for specific screening following activities that theoretically expose a person to infected blood such as body piercing and tattoos.

Among MSM, a detailed sexual history is warranted, with particular attention to sexual practices that would lead to mucosal damage (e.g., use of dilative sex toys), use of phosphodiesterase-5 inhibitors, illicit drug use during sex, sex causing anal bleeding, and group sex, as these were found to be associated with increased rates of acute HCV acquisition.[10]

A barrier to ascertaining risk factors for acute HCV is the underreporting of these behaviors to providers due to associated stigma.

Symptoms and Signs

Most patients are asymptomatic or minimally symptomatic from acute HCV. Some may report a flu-like illness, with or without jaundice, in the weeks prior to presentation; such history increases clinical suspicion for acute HCV but by itself is not diagnostic. On physical exam, jaundice may or may not be present, and there may be stigmata of other comorbidities (i.e., scars and infections of the skin associated with IDU), but the physical exam may be unrevealing or nonspecific.

Diagnostic Testing

Antibody Testing

The definitive way to diagnose new HCV infection is seroconversion in a person with previously documented seronegative status. Unfortunately, HCV antibodies alone are not an ideal measure of acute infection since they can remain undetectable for several weeks after initial infection and are therefore insensitive immediately following infection. Development of antibody titers can be further delayed in HIV-positive MSM, with a median time to seroconversion of 3 months.[11]

Past testing may be absent or results uncertain, and a positive antibody is not specific for acute infection as they remain elevated throughout the course of infection. Thus antibody testing cannot alone be used in this setting.

Aminotransferases and Bilirubin

Acute hepatitis is an indication for further screening, especially when risk factors are present. Elevations of alanine aminotransferase (ALT) are greater than aspartate aminotransferase (AST), and a cholestatic picture is rarely encountered. Jaundice and hyperbilirubinemia may accompany severe elevations of ALT in a small minority of cases. Seroconversion has been documented with minimal changes in liver function tests during the acute phase, and thus the absence of elevations does not exclude acute HCV infection. As the diagnosis of acute HCV needs to be done in a timely manner, rapid follow-up of elevated liver function tests is recommended even if the patient is asymptomatic.

Viral Load Testing

HCV RNA may be detectable as early as 1–2 weeks after infection, at times accompanied by a rise in ALT levels soon after that. Therefore, a detectable

HCV RNA with absence of anti-HCV antibodies (during the "seronegative window") is strongly suggestive of acute infection.

Both low viral titers (<10^5 IU/mL) and viral fluctuations (>1 log) are not common during the later phases of HCV infection and are thus suggestive of acute infection.[12] Serial HCV RNA testing may therefore be helpful for both diagnosis and to determine outcome (spontaneous clearance vs. persistence). Spontaneous clearance is also rare in the chronic phase of infection and can also suggest the acute phase. (Specific tests are covered in Chapter 4.)

HCV RNA is an important test that can help diagnose reinfection after viral clearance (as antibodies are already elevated from the first infection).

Other Testing

As acute HCV infection may be difficult to distinguish from other causes of acute hepatitis (especially on top of chronic HCV infection), tests for other causes of enzyme elevation are recommended (e.g., anti-HAV IgM, HBVSAg, and anti-HBV core IgM, abdominal ultrasound). If the patient is viremic and qualifies as a candidate for antiviral treatment, a HCV genotype is recommended. Genetic polymorphisms related to interleukin-28B (β subunit of IL-28, or interferon-λ-3) have been linked to both spontaneous and treatment-induced clearance. While this genetic test may help with prognosis, its utility in the acute setting has yet to be determined.

Treatment

Treatment for acute HCV infection is similar to that of chronic HCV infection and is highly effective. The question with treatment in the acute setting is the timing of treatment initiation, given the possibility of spontaneous clearance.

Because *symptomatic* acute HCV infection seems to be associated with a higher rate of spontaneous clearance of HCV, some authorities have suggested waiting a certain amount of time before initiating treatment in an attempt to avoid subjecting those patients most likely to spontaneously clear the virus to unnecessary treatment. Waiting up to 12 weeks in symptomatic patients to see if they clear the virus spontaneously before starting treatment is cost-effective, avoids unnecessary treatment for individuals who spontaneously clear HCV, and is associated with sustained virologic response on par with those starting treatment immediately.[13] For asymptomatic individuals, however, there are few data available to suggest the optimal timing of treatment initiation. Since these individuals are less likely to clear the virus spontaneously, it may be reasonable to start therapy immediately.

If the decision is made to delay immediate treatment, monitoring for up to 6 months is recommended to monitor for spontaneous clearance. If spontaneous clearance does not occur and treatment is initiated, recommended treatment is the same as that for chronic HCV infection. If the decision is made to initiate treatment during the acute infection period, monitoring HCV RNA for at least 12–16 weeks to allow for spontaneous clearance is recommended before starting treatment. Again, the recommended treatment is the same as that for chronic HCV infection, although preliminary trials suggest that shorter duration treatment may also be efficacious.

References

1. Centers for Disease Control. Surveillance for viral hepatitis—United States, 2014. https://www.cdc.gov/hepatitis/statistics/2014surveillance/commentary.htm#bkgrndC.

2. Zibbell JE, Iqbal K, Patel RC, et al. Increases in hepatitis C virus infection related to injection drug use among persons aged ≤30 years—Kentucky, Tennessee, Virginia, and West Virginia, 2006–2012. *MMWR*. 2015;64(17):453–458.

3. Massachusetts Department of Public Health, Bureau of Infectious Disease and Laboratory Sciences. Hepatitis C virus infection 2015 surveillance report. http://www.mass.gov/eohhs/gov/departments/dph/programs/id/. Published March 2016. Accessed January 28, 2017.

4. Broz D, Ouellet LJ. Racial and ethnic changes in heroin injection in the United States: implications for the HIV/AIDS epidemic. *Drug Alcohol Depend*. 2008;94(1):221–233.

5. Vogel M, Boesecke C, Rockstroh JK. Acute hepatitis C infection in HIV-positive patients. *Curr Opin Infect Dis*. 2011;24(1):1–6.

6. Maheshwari A, Ray S, Thuluvath PJ. Acute hepatitis C. *Lancet*. 2008;372(9635):321–332.

7. Grebely J, Page K, Sacks-Davis R, et al. The effects of female sex, viral genotype, and IL28B genotype on spontaneous clearance of acute hepatitis C virus infection. *Hepatology*. 2014;59(1):109–120.

8. Hagan H, Pouget ER, Des Jarlais DC, Lelutiu-Weinberger C. Meta-regression of hepatitis C virus infection in relation to time since onset of illicit drug injection: the influence of time and place. *Am J Epidemiol*. 2008;168(10):1099–1109.

9. Hagan H, Pouget ER, Des Jarlais DC. A systematic review and meta-analysis of interventions to prevent hepatitis C virus infection in people who inject drugs. *J Infect Dis*. 2011;204(1):74–83.

10. CDC. Sexual transmission of hepatitis C virus among HIV-infected men who have sex with men, New York City 2005. *MMWR*. 2011;60:945–950.

11. Thomson EC, Nastouli E, Main J, et al. Delayed anti-HCV antibody response in HIV-positive men acutely infected with HCV. *AIDS*. 2009;23(1):89–93.

12. McGovern BH, Birch CE, Bowen MJ, et al. Improving the diagnosis of acute hepatitis C virus infection with expanded viral load criteria. *Clin Infect Dis*. 2009;49(7):1051–1060.

13. Recommendations for testing, managing, and treating hepatitis C. http://hcvguidelines.org. Published September 2016. Accessed January 29, 2017.

Chapter 7

Chronic Hepatitis C

Rohit Satoskar and Tenzin Choden

Scope of the Problem

Hepatitis C virus (HCV) remains a global problem. It is estimated that the worldwide prevalence of HCV is as high as 3%, or 170 million individuals.[1] Prevalence estimates vary by region and are highest in Africa and Central and East Asia.[2] An estimated 14 million people in the Americas and 83 million people in Asia have chronic HCV. In the United States, the Centers for Disease Control and Prevention (CDC) estimate that between 2.7 and 3.9 million people are chronically infected with HCV. The majority of these cases are those born between 1945 and 1965 who were infected during the 1970s and 1980s, when infection rates were the highest. Prevalence of chronic hepatitis C is directly related to the previous incidence of acute hepatitis C, which varies depending on age and time.

Unfortunately, in the United States, the incidence of acute hepatitis C appears to be increasing: in 2014, 2,194 cases of acute HCV infection were reported to the CDC, with an incidence of 0.7 cases per 100,000 people, an increase from the 2010–2012 data. Because most cases of acute HCV are asymptomatic, leading to underascertainment and underreporting, this is likely an underrepresentation of the estimated 30,500 cases. In recent years, there has been an emerging epidemic of HCV infection among persons aged 20–29 years who are IV drug users, particularly in rural and suburban settings.[3] They now make up the subgroup with the highest reported incidence of acute hepatitis C in the United States.[4]

With these increases in the incidence of acute infection and subsequent chronic HCV infection, the incidences of cirrhosis with associated decompensation, hepatocellular carcinoma (HCC), and liver-related deaths are expected to increase over the next decade (Figure 7.1). As the prevalence of more advanced liver disease increases, the financial burden associated with chronic HCV will also increase. Total annual cost related to HCV in the United States was estimated at $6.5 billion in 2013 and is forecasted to increase to $9.1 billion in 2024.[5] The CDC estimates that there were almost 20,000 deaths with HCV as an underlying or contributing cause in the United States in 2014, and globally the World Health Organization (WHO) estimates that more than HCV-related 700,000 deaths occur every year.[6] HCV-related liver disease and complications remain the leading indication for liver transplantation in the United States and the world.

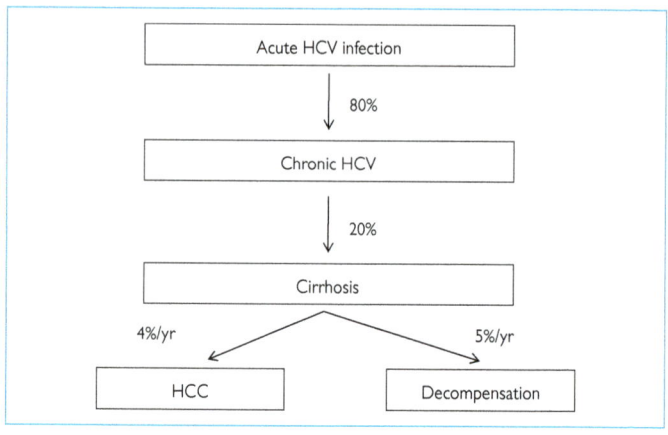

Figure 7.1 Natural history of HCV infection

Elimination of hepatitis C is an epidemiological challenge. Theoretically, it is feasible since the virus has no known nonhuman reservoir and there is a complete cure for an infected patient. Although the biology of the virus and treatment-based elimination are both promising, there are certain barriers. Hepatitis C remains largely asymptomatic and many of the heavily HCV-infected populations, such as IV drug users, are part of marginalized groups that are difficult to reach. Therefore, screening to identify HCV-positive patients as well as removing barriers to cure, such as restrictions on who can be treated, are paramount to the elimination endeavor.[7] Development of a vaccine for HCV will greatly help efforts at elimination.

Risk Factors and Screening

The most important risk factor for HCV infection is past or present injection drug use.[8] More than 60% of new HCV infections are found in patients who report injection drug use in the past 6 months. Additional risk factors are receipt of a blood transfusion before 1992, long-term hemodialysis, incarceration, being born to an HCV-infected mother, unregulated tattoos, and percutaneous exposures.

Most patients with chronic HCV are unaware of their infection. A risk-based approach requires that the patient both fully disclose risk factors as well as have knowledge about prior risk status. Since this risk-based approach can miss detecting a significant number of HCV-infected persons, the US Preventative Services Task Force (USPSTF) and the CDC now recommend a one-time screening of all persons born between 1945 and 1965.[9] In a study done by Smith et al. in 2011 examining anti-HCV antibody prevalence, more than 80% of anti-HCV positivity occurred among persons born from 1945 to 1965.[10] The USPSTF also recommends that persons with continued HCV risk factors should be screened periodically, although there is no current consensus on how often this screening should occur.

Presentation

The clinical presentation of chronic HCV depends largely on the stage of the underlying liver disease. There may be a wide range of presentations, from asymptomatic patients found to have abnormal alanine aminotransferase (ALT) levels to those who present with decompensated liver cirrhosis.[11]

Symptoms

The majority of patients found to have chronic hepatitis C do not exhibit specific symptoms. Of those with symptoms, the most common complaint is fatigue. Additional symptoms may include nausea, weight loss, arthralgia, or weakness. Less commonly, patients may present with extrahepatic manifestations of chronic HCV such as arthritis, renal dysfunction, autoimmune disorders, lichen planus, porphyria cutanea tarda, or leukocytoclastic vasculitis (Box 7.1).[12]

Laboratory Abnormalities

A positive anti-HCV antibody by second- or third-generation enzyme-linked immunosorbent assay (ELISA) has a greater than 90% positive predictive value in high-prevalence populations. Patients with a positive HCV

Box 7.1 Chronic HCV, Extrahepatic Manifestations/Associations

Dermatologic
Lichen planus
Porphyria cutanea tarda
Leukocytoclastic vasculitis
Raynaud's phenomenon

Rheumatologic
Arthritis/arthralgia
Myalgia

Hematologic
Essential mixed cryoglobulinemia
Monoclonal gammopathy
Lymphoma

Renal
Membranoproliferative nephritis

Other
Sicca syndrome
Uveitis
Neuropathy
Diabetes mellitus

antibody should undergo confirmatory testing of HCV infection. Most commonly, testing for serum HCV RNA detection by polymerase chain reaction (PCR) is performed. Patients who are immunocompromised or have end-stage renal disease on dialysis may not exhibit HCV antibodies even in the setting of chronic infection. In these populations, patients at risk should be tested for serum HCV RNA even in the absence of a positive HCV antibody test.

Differentiation between acute and chronic infection must be made on the basis of clinical presentation. Patients with a recent known exposure to HCV, high ALT level, clinical symptoms of acute hepatitis, and known previous normal ALT results should be considered for the possibility of acute HCV. The remainder of patients will likely have chronic HCV. Acute liver failure from HCV is rare.

Two-thirds of patients with chronic HCV will exhibit an elevated ALT level. The degree of elevation in ALT tends to vary over time. ALT levels do not correlate well with the severity of underlying liver histology. HCV genotyping should be performed in all patients with chronic HCV and may guide therapy.

Cirrhosis

The majority of morbidity and mortality in patients with chronic HCV results from the development of cirrhosis of the liver. Approximately 80% of patients with acute HCV infection will develop chronic disease.[13] Of the patients who develop chronic hepatitis C, up to 20% will eventually progress to cirrhosis of the liver; therefore, staging all patients with chronic hepatitis C is mandatory.[14]

In general, progression of disease occurs slowly, with a median time of 30 years for development of cirrhosis. Recent data based on the US National Health and Nutrition Examination Survey sample show that the prevalence of cirrhosis in patients with HCV infection has increased from 6.6% to 17% in the most recent era.[15] Factors associated with increased rates of fibrosis include longer duration of infection, alcohol consumption, age over 40 years at infection, male gender, elevated ALT level, diabetes, genotype 3, and coinfection with HIV (Box 7.2).[16] Patients with obesity and metabolic syndrome, who are more likely to have to hepatic steatosis, are also more prone to have progression of fibrosis in chronic HCV.[17] The use of lipid-lowering medications including statins is generally not contraindicated in this group.

Box 7.2 Risk Factors for Increased Fibrosis in Chronic HCV

Longer duration of infection
Alcohol consumption >50 g/day
Age >40 years at infection
Male gender
HIV coinfection
Steatosis
Genotype 3
Diabetes

Once cirrhosis has developed, if well compensated, 5-year survival ranges from 83% to 91%.[18] Decompensated disease including ascites, hepatic encephalopathy, jaundice, or variceal bleeding has an overall annual incidence rate of 3.9%.[19] Ascites is generally the most common presenting form of decompensation. Unfortunately, after decompensation, 5-year survival drops to 28–50%. Patients with cirrhosis should be cautioned against using both hepatotoxic and nephrotoxic drugs. They are also more susceptible to invasive pneumococcal infection and should receive early pneumococcal vaccination per CDC guidelines. Due to poor spontaneous survival rates, patients with decompensated cirrhosis should be considered for liver transplantation at centers with appropriate expertise.

In general, the complications of cirrhosis can be divided into those due to portal hypertension and those due to liver insufficiency or decreased synthetic dysfunction. Varices, variceal bleeding, ascites, spontaneous bacterial peritonitis, and hepatorenal syndrome are direct results of portal hypertension. Hepatic encephalopathy results from a combination of portal hypertension and impaired liver function. Other complications of cirrhosis include HCC and the liver–lung syndromes: hepatopulmonary syndrome and portopulmonary hypertension (Box 7.3).

Varices and Variceal Bleeding

Up to 50% of cirrhotic patients will have gastroesophageal varices at diagnosis. The prevalence of varices increases with the severity of underlying liver disease according to Child-Pugh score. Greater than 75% of patients who present with Child C cirrhosis will have gastroesophageal varices. Short-term mortality from acute variceal hemorrhage, while improved over the past two decades, remains high at about 30%. Because of the prevalence of varices in cirrhosis and the high risk of mortality associated with variceal bleeding, it is recommended that most patients undergo screening for varices with upper endoscopy.[20] Patients who have a liver stiffness measurement of less than 20 kPa and a platelet count of greater than 150,000/mm^3 are unlikely to have high-risk varices, and upper endoscopy may be avoidable in this group. If present, the size of varices at endoscopy is one of the greatest predictors of future bleeding. Patients with medium to large esophageal varices have a 30% risk of bleeding over 2 years. These patients should undergo primary prophylaxis of bleeding with a nonselective β-blocker or Carvedilol or with

---

Box 7.3 Complications of Cirrhosis

Variceal bleeding
Ascites
Spontaneous bacterial peritonitis
Jaundice
Hepatorenal syndrome
Hepatocellular carcinoma (HCC)
Hepatopulmonary syndrome
Portopulmonary hypertension
Hepatic encephalopathy
Protein-calorie malnutrition

serial endoscopic variceal ligation (EVL). Patients with small esophageal varices which have never bled but with other high-risk features including red signs or advanced liver disease (Child-Pugh C) should be placed on a nonselective β-blocker.

Hepatocellular Carcinoma

HCC is the fifth most common cancer worldwide in men and accounts for 5.6% of all cancers. The incidence of HCC has been rising since the early 1980s, and it is now the second leading cause of cancer-related mortality worldwide. There is significant geographic variation in the incidence of HCC, with highest rates in Asia and Sub-Saharan Africa. In the United States, while overall cancer death rates decreased between 2003 and 2013, liver cancer incidence rates have increased sharply (72%) and deaths from liver cancer increased at the highest rate.[21] HCV and liver cancer–associated death rates are highest among those born between 1945 and 1965. Overall, the 5-year survival rate of liver cancer is less than 17%. Eighty percent of HCC cases occur in patients with underlying cirrhosis of the liver.

Overall, chronic HCV infection accounts for up to 20% of HCC cases. The yearly incidence of HCC in patients with cirrhosis from all causes is 2–8%. While most cases of HCC in patients with chronic HCV occur in the setting of cirrhosis, there are also documented cases of HCC developing in HCV patients without cirrhosis. Data from HALT-C showed that this 5-year cumulative risk of developing HCC with bridging fibrosis was 4.1%. All patients with chronic HCV should be screened for HIV and HBV, since coinfection with HBV or HIV is associated with an increased risk of HCC. Those with HCV/HIV coinfection may have a 10- to 20-fold increased risk of HCC. Chronic HCV patients with porphyria cutanea tarda and alcohol consumption are also at increased risk of HCC. Patients with chronic HCV in the absence of cirrhosis who achieve a sustained virologic response (SVR) with treatment reduce their risk of developing HCC by more than 70% and have a 90% reduction in the risk of liver-related mortality and liver transplantation. Patients with HCV-related cirrhosis who are treated and cured of HCV should continue to have surveillance of HCC.[22]

Screening and Surveillance

Screening for cancers has now become routine practice in medicine. *Screening* is a public health service in which members of a defined population are offered a test to identify individuals who are likely to benefit from further testing or treatment aimed at reducing the risk of a disease or its complications. *Surveillance*, on the other hand, is the continuous monitoring of disease occurrence using the screening test within an at-risk population to achieve the same goals as screening. The utility of screening high-risk populations for HCC has been debated for many years, largely due to the lack of multiple randomized controlled trials. However, surveillance is widely accepted and applied.

According to the American Association for the Study of Liver Diseases (AASLD) guidelines, patients with underlying cirrhosis from chronic HCV should undergo surveillance for HCC with ultrasound every 6 months (Table 7.1).[23] Recent guidance from AASLD and the Infectious Disease Society of America also recommend surveillance in those with advanced fibrosis. Ultrasound has a sensitivity between 65% and 94% and a specificity of more than 90% when used for screening. A meta-analysis using 19 studies showed that ultrasound had a pooled sensitivity of 94% for detection of the majority of HCC tumors; however, it is less effective when detecting early-stage HCC (sensitivity of 63%).[24] This is likely due to the difficulty of detecting HCC on a cirrhotic background, which produces a coarse pattern on ultrasound. The use of ultrasound has also been criticized due to operator dependence and difficult visualization in patients who are obese. Computed tomography (CT) and magnetic resonance imaging (MRI) have demonstrated excellent specificity when used for diagnosis but have not been well studied in the setting of surveillance. While many centers use CT or MRI to screen for HCC, it is also not clear that this approach is cost-effective, and most liver societies continue to recommend ultrasound as the imaging of choice for HCC screening. The use of tumor markers, including α-fetoprotein (AFP), Des-γ-carboxy prothrombin (DCP), and prothrombin induced by vitamin K absence II (PIVKA II), has been omitted from the AASLD and EASL practice guidelines due to the lack of strong data to support this practice.[25] Despite this, other societies continue to recommend the use of tumor markers, and many US centers continue to test for them.[26]

Both AASLD and EASL recommend surveillance for patients with chronic HCV and bridging fibrosis without documented cirrhosis. Most centers continue to screen these patients due to the increased risk of HCC, as shown in the HALT-C studies, as well as the possibility of understaging with biopsy. Screening at more frequent intervals (i.e., 3 months) has not been shown to be more effective. Prolonging the surveillance intervals to annually from 6 months has shown a decrease in pooled sensitivity from 70% to 50%.[27]

Standard recall procedures should be in place for those found to have an abnormality on screening. Patients with an abnormality on screening ultrasound should have evaluation with a four-phase dynamic MRI or CT to more definitively characterize the lesion. If the findings are characteristic of HCC

Table 7.1 Recommendations for hepatocellular carcinoma surveillance in high-risk patients

American Association for the Study of Liver Diseases (AASLD)	European Association for the Study of the Liver (EASL)	Asian Pacific Association for the Study of the Liver (APASL)	National Comprehensive Cancer Network (NCCN)
Ultrasound every 6 months	Ultrasound every 6 months	Ultrasound and AFP every 6 months	Ultrasound and AFP every 6 months

on either study, the lesion should be managed as such. If atypical on both studies, biopsy may be considered to reach a definitive diagnosis.

Various therapies are available for the treatment of HCC. Treatment should be pursued in conjunction with a liver transplant center or a care provider experienced in the management of HCC. Choice of treatment depends on the degree of underlying liver disease, stage of HCC, comorbidities, and patient preference. For early HCC, "curative" measures such as liver transplantation and hepatic resection may be considered. Transarterial chemoembolization (TACE), radiofrequency ablation (RFA), radioembolization, and other liver-directed therapies may be considered in patients who are not surgical candidates or as a bridge to transplantation. For patients with advanced disease, systemic chemotherapy, as with sorafenib, may be considered.

References

1. World Health Organization (WHO). Hepatitis C: Fact sheet. http://www.who.int/mediacentre/factsheets/fs164/en/. Updated July 2016. Accessed January 24, 2017.

2. Lavanchy, D. The global burden of hepatitis C. *Liver Int*. 2014;29(Suppl 1):74–81.

3. John-Baptiste A, Krahn M, Heathcote J, et al. The natural history of hepatitis C infection acquired through injection drug use: Meta-analysis and meta-regression. *J Hepatol*. 2010;53(2):245–251.

4. Suryaprasad AG, White JZ, Xu F, et al. Emerging epidemic of hepatitis C virus infections among young nonurban persons who inject drugs in the United States, 2006–2012. *Clin Infect Dis*. 2014;59(10):1411–1419.

5. Razavi H, Elkhoury AC, Elbasha E, et al. Chronic hepatitis C virus (HCV) disease burden and cost in the United States. *Hepatology*. 2013;57(6):2164–2170.

6. Centers for Disease Control and Prevention (CDC). Hepatitis C FAQs for health professionals: Overview and statistics. https://www.cdc.gov/hepatitis/hcv/hcvfaq.htm#. Accessed January 24, 2017.

7. Moyer V. Screening for hepatitis C virus infection in adults: US Preventive Services Task Force recommendation statement. *Ann Intern Med*. 2013;159:349–357.

8. Committee on a National Strategy for the Elimination of Hepatitis B and C; Board on Population Health and Public Health Practice; Health and Medicine Division; National Academies of Sciences, Engineering, and Medicine. The elimination of hepatitis C. In Buckley GJ, Strom BL, eds. *Eliminating the public health problem of hepatitis B and C in the United States: Phase one report*. Washington, DC: National Academies Press (US);2016:83–134. https://www.ncbi.nlm.nih.gov/books/NBK368067/

9. AASLD-IDSA. Recommendations for testing, managing, and treating hepatitis C. http://www.hcvguidelines.org. Accessed January 24, 2017.

10. Smith BD, Patel N, Beckett GA, et al. Hepatitis C virus antibody prevalence, correlates and predictors among persons born from 1945 through 1965, United States, 1999–2008 [Abstract]. *Hepatology*. 2011;54:4(Suppl 1):554A–555A.

11. Westbrook RH, Dusheiko G. Natural history of hepatitis C. *J Hepatol*. 2014;61(1 Suppl):S58–S68.

12. El-Serag HB, Hampel H, Yeh C, et al. Extrahepatic manifestations of hepatitis C among United States male veterans. *Hepatology*. 2002;36(6):1439–1445.

13. Gordon SC, Lamerato LE, Rupp LB, et al. Prevalence of cirrhosis in hepatitis C patients in the Chronic Hepatitis Cohort Study (CHeCS): A retrospective and prospective observational study. *Am J Gastroenterol*. 2015;110(8):1169–1177.

14. Hu KQ, Tong MJ. The long-term outcomes of patients with compensated hepatitis C virus-related cirrhosis and history of parenteral exposure in the United States. *Hepatology*. 1999;29(4):1311–1316.

15. Udompap P, Mannalithara A, Heo NY, et al. Increasing prevalence of cirrhosis among US adults aware or unaware of their chronic hepatitis C virus infection. *J Hepatol*. 2016;64(5):1027–1032.

16. Kanwal F, Kramer J, Ilyas J, et al. HCV genotype 3 is associated with an increased risk of cirrhosis and hepatocellular cancer in a national sample of US Veterans with HCV. *Hepatology*. 2014;60(1):98–105.

17. Poynard T, Bedossa P, Opolon P. Natural history of liver fibrosis progression in patients with chronic hepatitis C. The OBSVIRC, METAVIR, CLINIVIR, and DOSVIRC groups. *Lancet*. 1997;349(9055):825–832.

18. Fattovich G, Giustina G, Degos F, et al. Morbidity and mortality in compensated cirrhosis type C: A retrospective follow-up study of 384 patients. *Gastroenterology*. 1997;112(2):463–472.

19. Liang TJ, Rehermann B, Seeff LB, et al. Pathogenesis, natural history, treatment, and prevention of hepatitis C. *Ann Intern Med*. 2000;132(4):296–305.

20. Garcia-Tsao G, Abraldes J, Berzigotti A, et al. Portal hypertensive bleeding in cirrhosis: Risk stratification, diagnosis, and management. 2016 practice guidance by the American Association for the study of liver diseases. *Hepatology*. 2016;65(1):310–335.

21. Ryerson AB, Eheman C, Altekruse S, et al. Annual report to the nation on the status of cancer, 1975–2012, featuring the increasing incidence of liver cancer. *Cancer*. 2016;122:1312–1337.

22. Bruix J, Sherman M. Management of hepatocellular carcinoma: An update. http://www.aasld.org/sites/default/files/guideline_documents/HCCUpdate2010.pdf. Accessed March 3, 2017.

23. Ghany MG, Strader DB, Thomas DL, et al. Diagnosis, management, and treatment of hepatitis C: An update. *Hepatology*. 2009;49(4):1335–1374.

24. Singal A, Volk ML, Waljee A, et al. Meta-analysis: Surveillance with ultrasound for early-stage hepatocellular carcinoma in patients with cirrhosis. *Aliment Pharmacol Ther*. 2009;30:3747.

25. European Association for the Study of the Liver (EASL). Management of hepatocellular carcinoma: EASL-EORTC clinical practice guidelines. http://www.easl.eu/research/our-contributions/clinical-practice-guidelines/detail/management-of-hepatocellular-carcinoma-easl-eortc-clinical-practice-guidelines/report/4. Accessed January 23, 2017.

26. Omata M, Lesmana LA, Tateishi R, et al. Asian Pacific Association for the Study of the Liver consensus recommendations on hepatocellular carcinoma. *Hepatol Int*. 2010;4(2):439–474.

27. Trinchet JC, Chaffaut C, Bourcier V, et al. Ultrasonographic surveillance of hepatocellular carcinoma in cirrhosis: A randomized trial comparing 3- and 6-month periodicities. *Hepatology*. 2011;54:1987–1997.

Chapter 8

Extrahepatic Manifestations of Hepatitis C

Suzanne Robertazzi and Anjana A. Pillai

Introduction

Since the identification of the hepatitis C virus (HCV), several associations have been discovered between the virus and a variety of extrahepatic clinical manifestations (Box 8.1). Studies report that up to 40% of patients with chronic hepatitis C infection have at least one extrahepatic manifestation.[1,2] Extrahepatic manifestations have been theorized to trigger clinical disease in numerous organ systems, causing renal, vascular, endocrine, rheumatologic, dermatologic, neurologic, and ophthalmologic involvement.[3] While the exact mechanisms triggering these extrahepatic manifestations in patients with HCV is not always well-defined, there are several associations that have a well-established causal relationship, and symptomatic improvement is seen with viral eradication. This review will highlight three extrahepatic manifestations that have well-documented correlations with hepatitis C viremia: mixed cryoglobulinemia, B-cell lymphoma, and porphyria cutanea tarda (PCT). With the availability of all-oral direct-acting antiviral regimens, the impact of a sustained virologic response on these extrahepatic manifestations should significantly improve hepatic and extrahepatic morbidity and mortality.

Mixed Cryoglobulinemia

Case: 55-year-old Caucasian woman with genotype 1b hepatitis C was evaluated for a new purpuric rash on her bilateral lower extremities and significant proteinuria. Patient had a recent liver biopsy that showed chronic hepatitis C with grade 3 inflammation and stage 3 fibrosis. Her HCV viral load was 212,785 IU/mL. Her cryoglobulin screen was positive. A renal biopsy revealed "cryoglobulinemic hepatitis C-associated membranoproliferative glomerulonephritis." Patient was started on direct-acting antiviral (DAA) therapy with fixed-dose ledipasvir/sofosbuvir for 12 weeks. Her proteinuria and rash resolved after 8 weeks of treatment. She had a 12-week sustained virologic response (SVR12) and has had no further recurrence of her vasculitis.

> **Box 8.1 Extrahepatic Manifestations of Chronic Hepatitis C Infection**
>
> - Mixed cryoglobulinemia
> - Non-Hodgkin's lymphoma
> - Membranoproliferative glomerulonephritis
> - Leukocytoclastic vasculitis
> - Porphyria cutanea tarda
> - Lichen planus
> - Thyroid abnormalities
> - Diabetes mellitus
> - Sicca syndrome
> - Autoantibodies
> - Peripheral neuropathy
> - Neurocognitive dysfunction
> - Idiopathic pulmonary fibrosis

Mixed cryoglobulinemia (MC) is the most common extrahepatic manifestation associated with HCV and is characterized by the deposition of circulating immune complexes in the small vessels of various organs, leading to a systemic vasculitis. Cryoglobulin complexes were first described in the literature in 1966, by Meltzer and Franklin, in a group of patients who expressed the triad of purpura, arthralgia, and weakness without an identifiable underlying disease process.[4] MC is believed to be an HCV-related lymphoproliferative disorder.

Cryoglobulins are circulating immunoglobulins that precipitate when serum is cooled below core body temperature and resolubilize when warmed. They are classified into three subtypes. Type I is composed of monoclonal immunoglobulins and frequently associated with hematologic malignancies. Type II is composed of polyclonal IgG and monoclonal IgM, and type III is composed of polyclonal IgG and polyclonal IgM.[5] HCV is primarily seen with type II MC.

MC can involve multiple organ systems, affecting the small and medium-sized vessels of the skin, peripheral nerves, kidneys, and salivary and lacrimal glands.[2,5] Serum cryoglobulins have been detected in 40–60% of patients with HCV,[6,7] yet only 10–15% of these patients develop symptomatic MC.[8] The reason for this discrepancy remains unknown. In addition, patients with MC have a higher incidence of advanced fibrosis and cirrhosis compared to patients without detectable cryoglobulins.[6,9]

Because of its variable presentation, there are no standardized criteria for the diagnosis of MC. Typically, the diagnosis is made when patients present with clinical manifestations in the setting of positive serum cryoglobulins. An elevated rheumatoid factor and reduced C4 counts may also be useful to confirm the diagnosis.[2] Some patients may show clinical symptoms of MC without having detectable serum cryoglobulins.[2] Improper collection and transport of samples are the most common reasons for a false-negative cryoglobulin screen.

The most common manifestation of HCV-associated MC is palpable purpura of the lower extremities, where venous stasis favors the precipitation of cryoglobulins (Figure 8.1). This rash is often preceded by paresthesias.[1,5] Additional symptoms include arthralgias, fatigue, and weakness. Purpuric lesions may progress to large chronic necrotic ulcers. Membranoproliferative glomerulonephritis, the renal manifestation of MC, can occur in up to one-third of patients. Findings range from arterial hypertension, isolated proteinuria (usually in the nonnephrotic range), microscopic hematuria, and mild renal insufficiency to progressive renal failure.[2,5] The presence of renal involvement is a negative prognostic factor in patients with MC. Neurologic involvement can result in painful paresthesias and concomitant weakness leading to a foot or wrist drop.[5]

The most effective treatment for MC is eradication of the HCV infection. The American Association for the Study of Liver Disease (AASLD) HCV Guidance, Recommendations for Testing, Managing and Treating Hepatitis C include the use of one of many HCV DAA agent combinations as first-line treatment. The use of ribavirin (RBV) is recommended in special patient populations.[10] Prior to the use of DAAs, first-line therapy for HCV treatment consisted of standard-dose pegylated interferon (PEG-IFN) and RBV with the option to extend treatment to 48 weeks for genotypes 2/3 and 72 weeks for genotypes 1/4, with evidence of symptomatic improvement.[11] Gragnani et al.[12] conducted a multicenter prospective study looking at the effectiveness of different sofosbuvir-containing DAA regimens in the treatment of patients with HCV-associated MC. Of the 44 patients enrolled, 100% achieved a SVR24. All 44 patients had an overall improvement in their vasculitis, with 77% of the patients having a complete response, and 23% of the patients having a partial response. The investigators did note that peripheral neuropathy and sicca syndrome did persist in some patients despite achieving SVR24. In addition, two patients included in this cohort did receive rituximab in addition to the use of DAAs.[12]

Rituximab is a chimeric monoclonal antibody against the protein CD20, which is primarily found on the surface of B cells. Rituximab is generally safe and well tolerated.[13,14] Some experts recommend the use of rituximab followed by the initiation of antiviral therapy in patients with severe symptoms.[15]

Short courses of low-dose corticosteroids may be considered to control vasculitic flares in patients prior to the initiation of antiviral therapy or if antiviral therapy is unsuccessful. Corticosteroids are not recommended for continuous suppressive therapy given their deleterious side effects, including enhancing HCV replication.[13]

Finally, although data are limited, in patients with severe manifestations of MC, including severe vasculitis, plasmapheresis in conjunction with rituximab can be considered as a second-line option with variable success.[16]

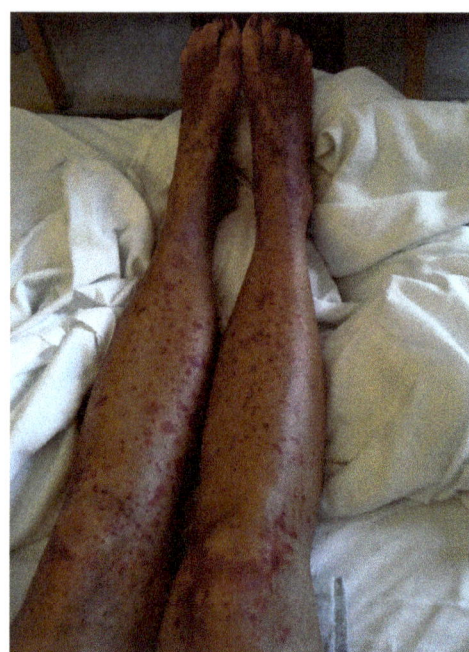

Figure 8.1 Leukocytoclastic vasculitis of lower extremities in patient with mixed cryoglobulinemia

B-Cell Lymphoma

Case: 68-year-old Hispanic woman with genotype 2 hepatitis C and stage 1 fibrosis on biopsy was admitted for abdominal pain and found to have anemia. A CT scan of the abdomen and pelvis was noncontributory. She underwent a bone marrow biopsy, which was consistent with a B-cell lymphoproliferative disorder. She also underwent a renal biopsy for acute renal failure with proteinuria and hematuria. Her renal biopsy also confirmed focal kidney involvement by a low-grade B-cell lymphoma. She was started on treatment with 12 weeks of daclatasvir and sofosbuvir and had a SVR12. Her lymphoma was found to be in remission without any evidence of malignancy on repeat bone marrow biopsy.

HCV, in addition to its hepatotropic properties, has known tropism for peripheral lymphocytes. It has been shown that the HCV envelope protein E2 binds to B lymphocytes via the tetraspanin CD81. This interaction is believed to lower the activation threshold of these cells, leading to chronic antigenic stimulation. This subsequently may lead to polyclonal B-cell expansion, progression to autonomous B-cell proliferation, immune dysregulation, and malignant transformation leading to the development of malignant lymphoma.[11,17] Another theory is that HCV induces mutagenesis, which leads to prolonged B-cell survival and eventual malignant transformation. Genetic and environmental factors are also believed to play a key role in the formation of B-cell lymphoma. Although the exact mechanism remains unclear, there is an undeniably strong link between HCV and B-cell lymphomas.

HCV viremia has been reported in up to 35% of patients with B-cell lymphoma, and almost 90% of non-Hodgkin's lymphoma (NHL) patients have detectable cryoglobulins.[18] MC patients have an estimated 35 times higher risk of NHL compared to the general population.[19] Approximately 8–10% of patients with HCV-associated MC will progress to a high-grade lymphoma.[2] Marginal-zone lymphoma appears to be the most frequently encountered low-grade B-cell lymphoma in HCV patients.[20] Among these there is an especially strong association between HCV and mucosa-associated lymphoid tissue (MALT) lymphoma.[1] Additionally, approximately 65% of HCV-related lymphomas have extranodal involvement, particularly in the salivary glands and the liver, compared to only 19% of non–HCV-related lymphomas.[20]

Antiviral therapy is a reasonable approach to the treatment of patients with low-grade HCV-associated lymphoma. PEG IFN-based treatments can lead to regression of these low-grade lymphomas after viral clearance.[20] The data for the use of DAAs are very limited, and only a few case reports of lymphoma regression have been published.[21] However, this is not the case with intermediate or high-grade lymphomas, where systemic chemotherapy remains the mainstay of treatment.[22] The use of rituximab as monotherapy or in combination with antiviral therapy and/or chemotherapy is also being studied. Small studies have shown successful use of rituximab monotherapy as first-line therapy for HCV-related indolent B-cell lymphoma.[23] Currently there are no recommendations for the use of DAAs in the treatment of HCV-associated lymphoma.

Porphyria Cutanea Tarda

Case: 49-year-old Caucasian man with newly diagnosed genotype 2b hepatitis C presented to clinic with a blistering rash on both of his hands. He was initially treated by his primary care physician with cortisone cream, which did not provide any relief. He was referred to a dermatologist, who gave him the diagnosis of PCT. His physical exam revealed numerous purple lesions on both his hands. There were no other lesions found on his body. Of note, laboratory values showed a significantly elevated ferritin of 1,508, negative cryoglobulin screen, and a HCV viral load of 413,852 IU/ mL. His total plasma porphyrins and 24-hour urine porphyrins were markedly elevated. A liver biopsy showed chronic hepatitis with mild chronic inflammatory activity and stage 1 fibrosis. Iron stain showed 2–3$^+$ iron in both hepatocytes and Kupffer cells. Therapeutic phlebotomy was initiated for his elevated ferritin, with subsequent normalization of his levels and improvement of his skin lesions. Antiviral therapy with fixed-dose sofosbuvir and velpatasvir for 12 weeks was started shortly afterward. He subsequently attained a SVR12. He did not have any further recurrence of his skin lesions.

PCT is a disorder characterized by reduced activity of uroporphyrinogen decarboxylase, an enzyme in the heme biosynthetic pathway. It is the most common of the porphyrias. It is associated with skin fragility, bullae formation, hypertrichosis of light-exposed areas, hyperpigmentation, scleromoid changes, dystrophic calcifications with ulcerations, scarring, alopecia, and onycholysis.[3,24] These lesions occur due to the photosensitizing effect of porphyrins that accumulate in the skin.

The exact effect of HCV on PCT is unknown but is believed to be related to HCV-induced hepatic iron overload. Development of PCT likely requires a combination of genetic, infectious, and environmental factors. HCV is the most common viral infection associated with PCT. In the United States alone, approximately 56% of patients with PCT have HCV, as opposed to only 2% of the general population.[24,25]

The diagnosis of PCT is based on increased urocarboxyl porphyrins and heptacarboxyporphyrins in the urine in addition to elevated liver function tests, ferritin, and serum iron.[25] A 24-urine porphyrin level of more than 2 micromoles suggests extensive liver accumulation of porphyrin. Liver biopsy findings include increased intracellular porphyrins or red fluorescence of biopsy tissue with long-wave ultraviolet light scans.[24]

Physical exam findings include erythema, skin fragility, bullae, erosions, and hypertrichosis. Blisters, vesicles, and milia are seen on the dorsal surface of the extremities, especially the hands and other photo-exposed areas.[3,25]

Treatment consists of lifestyle modifications, including sun avoidance or judicious use of sun block and protective clothing.[3] Therapeutic phlebotomy can be used to lower serum ferritin levels, which typically requires twice-weekly treatments for 2–3 months. Resolution of blisters is often seen in the first few months; however, reduction in skin fragility may take up to 9 months, and normalization of porphyrin concentrations may take over a year.[24] There are a few case reports using DAAs in the treatment of HCV-associated PCT. These case reports show great promise and support the resolution of PCT with the achievement of SVR.[26] Therapeutic phlebotomy should be considered prior to DAA treatment, with careful consideration prior to using phlebotomy in conjunction with RBV as the combination can lead to severe anemia. Currently, there are no standardized trials to determine the appropriate timing between discontinuing phlebotomy and starting antiviral therapy. Several case reports have shown the resolution of PCT once a SVR has been achieved.[27]

Conclusion

It is important to consider a multidisciplinary approach to treating patients with extrahepatic manifestations of chronic hepatitis C infection. These coexisting disease entities can add to the complexity of antiviral therapy, and the additional input from rheumatology, dermatology, nephrology, and oncology can help guide treatment and manage added side effects.

There is limited data using DAAs in the conditions described herein, but the current recommendations by the AASLD stress the importance of treating all patients with HCV. The favorable side-effect profile of the DAAs has increased the tolerability of treatment along with an increase in SVR rates. If patients with HCV can be treated earlier in their disease course, this can possibly decrease the number of patients who develop extrahepatic manifestations of HCV, thus improving patient quality of life.

References

1. Meyer D, Bodenheimer H. Extrahepatic manifestations of chronic hepatitis C infection. In: Shetty K, Wu G, eds. *Clinical gastroenterology: chronic viral hepatitis*. New York: Humana Press;2009:135–157.

2. Zignego AL, Craxì A. Extrahepatic manifestations of hepatitis C virus infection. *Clin Liver Dis*. 2008;12(3):611–636.

3. Sterling R, Bralow P. Extrahepatic manifestations of hepatitis C virus. *Curr Gastroenterol Rep*. 2006;8:53–59.

4. Meltzer M, Franklin EC. Cryoglobulinemia—a study of twenty-nine patients. I. IgG and IgM cryoglobulins and factors affecting cryoprecipitability. *Am J Med*. 1966;40(6):828–836.

5. Charles E, Dustin L. Hepatitis C virus-induced cryoglobulinemia. *Int Soc Nephrol*. 2009;76:818–824.

6. Lunel F, Musset L, Cacoub P, et al. Cryoglobulinemia in chronic liver diseases: role of hepatitis C virus and liver damage. *Gastroenterology*. 1994;106: 1291–1300.

7. Pawlotsky JM, Ben Yahia M, et al. Immunological disorders in C virus chronic active hepatitis: a prospective case-control study. *Hepatology*. 1994;19:841–848.

8. Saadoun D, Landau DA, Calabrese LH, Cacoub PP. Hepatitis C-associated mixed cryoglobulinaemia: a crossroad between autoimmunity and lymphoproliferation. *Rheumatology*. 2007;46:1234–1242.

9. Kayali Z, Buckwold VE, Zimmerman B, Schmidt WN. Hepatitis C, cryoglobulinemia, and cirrhosis: a meta-analysis. *Hepatology*. 2002;36(4):978–985.

10. AASLD-IDSA. Recommendations for testing, managing, and treating hepatitis C. www.hcvguidelines.org. Accessed on February 2, 2017.

11. Zignego A, Giannini C, Ferri C. Hepatitis C virus-related lymphopro-liferative disorders: an overview. *World J Gastroenterol*. 2007;13(17):2467–2478.

12. Gragnani L, et al. Prospective study of guideline-tailored therapy with direct-acting antivirals for hepatitis C virus associated mixed cryoglobulinemia. *Hepatology*. 2016;64(5):1473–1482.

13. Pietrogrande M, et al. Recommendations for the management of mixed cryoglobulinemia syndrome in hepatitis C virus-infected patients. *Autoimmun Rev*. 2011;10:444–454.

14. Saadoun D, Delluc A, Piette J, Cacoub P. Treatment of hepatitis c-associated mixed cryoglobulinemia vasculitis. *Curr Opin Rheumatol*. 2008;20:23–28.

15. Muchtar E, Magen H, Gertz M. How I treat cryoglobulinemia. *Blood J.* 2017;129(3):289–298

16. Emery JS, Kuczynski M, La D, et al. Efficacy and safety of direct acting antivirals for the treatment of mixed cryoglobulinemia. *Am J Gastoenterol.* 2017. doi: 10.1038/ajg.2017.49

17. Medina J, García-Buey L, Moreno-Otero R. Hepatitis C virus-related extrahepatic disease—aetiopathogenesis and management. *Aliment Pharmacol Ther.* 2004;20(2):129–141.

18. Galossi A, Guarisco R, Bellis L, Puoti, C. Extrahepatic manifestations of chronic HCV infection. *J Gastrointestin Liver Dis.* 2007;16:65–73.

19. Monti G, Pioltelli P, Saccardo F, et al. Incidence and characteristics of non-Hodgkin lymphomas in a multicenter case file of patients with hepatitis C virus-related symptomatic mixed cryoglobulinemias. *Arch Intern Med.* 2005;165(1):101–105.

20. Viswanatha D, Dogan A. Hepatitis C virus and lymphoma. *J Clin Pathol.* 2007;60:1378–1383.

21. Galati G, Rampa L, Vespasiani-Gentilucci U, et al. Hepatitis C and double-hit B cell lymphoma successfully treated by antiviral therapy. *World J Hepatol.* 2016;8(29):1244–1250.

22. Gisbert JP, Garcia-Buey L, Pajares JM, et al. Systematic review: regression of lymphoproliferative disorders after treatment for hepatitis C infection. *Aliment Pharmacol Ther.* 2005;21:653–662.

23. Hainsworth JD, Litchy S, Burris HA, III, et al. Rituximab as first-line and maintenance therapy for patients with indolent non-Hodgkin's lymphoma. *J Clin Oncol.* 2002;20:4261–4267.

24. Dienhart P, Sterling R. Management of hepatitis C virus in patients with porphyria cutanea tarda. *Curr Hepat Rep.* 2005;4:104–111.

25. Rebora A. Skin diseases associated with hepatitis C virus: facts and controversies. *Clin Dermatol.* 2010;28:489–496.

26. Tong Y, Song Y, Tyring, S. Resolution of porphyria cutanea tarda in patients with hepatitis C following ledipasvir-sofosbuvir combination therapy. *JAMA Dermatol.* 2016;152(12):1393–1395.

27. Azim J, McCurdy H, Moseley R. Porphyria cutanea tarda as a complication of therapy for chronic hepatitis C. *World J Gastroenterol.* 2008;14:5913–5915.

Feeney E, Chung R. Antiviral treatment of hepatitis C. *Br Med J.* 2014;348:3308.

Kohli A, Shaffer A, Serman A, Kottilil, S. Treatment of hepatitis C: a systemic review. *JAMA.* 2014;312(6):631–640.

Viganoi A, et al. The association of cryoglobulinaemia with sustained virological response in patients with chronic hepatitis C. *J Viral Hepatol.* 2011;18:e91–e98.

Wang X, Pillai A. Extrahepatic manifestations of chronic hepatitis C infection: a review and update. *Curr Hepatol Rep.* 2016;15:150–157.

Chapter 9

Treatment of Hepatitis C Genotypes 1, 4, 5, 6

Ramakrishna Behara and Steven L. Flamm

Introduction

Chronic hepatitis C virus (HCV) infection is a worldwide scourge and is a major cause of cirrhosis and hepatocellular carcinoma. It is the leading cause of liver transplantation in the Western world. HCV is characterized by six different genotypes. In the United States, HCV genotype 1 (GT1) accounts for approximately 75% of all HCV infections. HCV genotypes 2 (GT2) and 3 (GT3) are observed less frequently in the United States, although GT3 is common in other areas of the world. HCV genotype 4 (GT4), a genotype prevalent in Egypt, is uncommonly seen in the United States. Genotype 5 (GT5), observed in South Africa, and genotype 6 (GT6), seen in South-East Asia, are rarely encountered in the United States.

Because of the high prevalence of GT1, investigation of therapeutic regimens for HCV has focused on GT1. In the past, GT1 was the most difficult to cure with pegylated interferon-α (PEG-IFNα)–based regimens. However, with the advent of direct-acting antiviral agents (DAAs), GT1 patients are now among the easiest to achieve sustained virologic response (SVR).[1]

This chapter addresses current treatment recommendations for HCV GT1, 4, 5, and 6. However, it should be noted that new regimens are approved frequently and that therapeutic options continue to evolve rapidly. For that reason, the American Association for the Study of Liver Diseases (AASLD) and the Infectious Diseases Society of America (IDSA) have developed frequently updated guidance recommendations that are available online (www.hcvguidelines.org) and help providers make appropriate treatment decisions on behalf of their patients.

Older Regimens for GT1

PEG IFN/RBV

Before 2011, PEG-IFNα + ribavirin (RBV) therapy was the standard therapeutic regimen for HCV GT1. However, therapy was complicated by many side effects. Many patients had contraindications to the regimen and could not be treated. Others started therapy and could not tolerate the medications. Even when GT1 patients were able to take PEG-IFN and RBV for 48 weeks, fewer than one-half of patients were able to achieve SVR.[2,3]

PEG-IFN, RBV, and Protease Inhibitor

The first DAA agents, boceprevir and telaprevir (NS3/4 serine protease inhibitors [PIs]), were approved in 2011 in combination with PEG-IFN for GT1. SVR rates increased as compared with PEG-IFN and RBV alone, as revealed in multiple randomized controlled trials.[4–6] However, therapy was still complicated by contraindications to therapy and poor tolerability. Hence, non–PEG-IFN–based regimens were sought.

Newer Regimens for GT1

DAAs

A better understanding of the HCV genome has led to specific targeted therapy toward multiple nonstructural proteins of HCV. Three main targets exist, with the ultimate goal of disrupting viral replication and facilitating clearance of the virus. The NS3/4A PI class mentioned earlier has expanded to include glecaprevir, voxilaprevir, grazoprevir, paritaprevir, and simeprevir. The NS5A inhibitors include pibrentasvir, daclatasvir, elbasvir, ledipasvir, ombitasvir, and velpatasvir. Finally, the NS5B RNA-dependent RNA PIs can be split into two separate classes: nucleotide PIs (NPIs) (e.g., sofosbuvir), and non-nucleoside PIs (NNPIs) (e.g., dasabuvir). Clinical trials with combinations of these medications are discussed in Chapter 14.

Current Treatment Options for GT1

There are multiple all-oral fixed-dose combinations (FDC) (ledipasvir/sofosbuvir, sofosbuvir/velpatasvir, sofosbuvir/velpatasvir/voxilaprevir, paritaprevir/ritonavir/ombitasvir with dasabuvir, glecaprevir/pibrentasvir, and elbasvir/grazoprevir) and other combination regimens (sofosbuvir/simeprevir and sofosbuvir/daclatasvir) that have been approved to treat HCV GT1.

In general, regimens have similar efficacy and excellent safety profiles. Issues that dictate which regimens or how various regimens are used include GT1 subtype (1a vs. 1b), the presence of absence of cirrhosis, prior treatment exposure, baseline viral load and presence of baseline NS5A resistance-associated substitutions (RASs), potential drug–drug interactions (DDIs), potential contraindications for ribavirin, and the presence of renal insufficiency or decompensated cirrhosis. The AASLD/IDSA guidance documents prioritize RBV-free shorter duration therapies when available. In the presence of renal failure, sofosbuvir-based regimens are not recommended (glomerular filtration rate [GFR] <30, including dialysis). PI-containing regimens are contraindicated in patients with decompensated cirrhosis.

Table 9.1 Overview of drug classes and genotype

Drug Class	Genotype Covered (1, 4, 5, 6)
Elbasvir/Grazoprevir	1, 4
Ledipasvir/Sofosbuvir	1, 4, 5,6
Paritaprevir/Ritonavir/Ombitasvir plus Dasabuvir +/− weight-based Ribavirin	1, 4 (without Dasabuvir)
Simeprevir/Sofosbuvir	1
Sofosbuvir/Velpatasvir, Sofosbuvir/Velpatasvir/Voxilaprevir, Glecaprevir/Pibrentasvir	Pan-Genotypic
Daclatasvir/Sofosbuvir	1

Data on special populations of HCV subjects including HIV-HCV coinfected patients, patients with severe renal insufficiency or on dialysis, and patients with decompensated cirrhosis are discussed in other chapters.

Treatment Naïve or Experienced (PEG-IFN) Noncirrhotic GT1

Numerous treatment options exist with similar efficacy (Table 9.1, Box 9.1, Box 9.2). These include fixed-dose combinations of ledipasvir/sofosbuvir (LDV/SOF), paritaprevir/ritonavir/ombitasvir with dasabuvir (PRoD) +/− RBV, simeprevir/sofosbuvir (SIM/SOF), elbasvir/grazoprevir, sofosbuvir/velpatasvir (SOF/VEL), daclatasvir/sofosbuvir (DAC/SOF), and glecaprevir/pibrentasvir (GLE/PIB). In fact, for treatment-naïve GT1 patients without cirrhosis who have a baseline viral load of less than 6 million and are not HIV coinfected, a truncated course of 8 weeks of therapy could be considered. Currently, NS5A RAS testing is recommended for GT1a patients considering elbasvir/grazoprevir. If impactful RAS are found to be present (NS5A resistance-associated polymorphisms at amino acid positions 28, 30, 31, or 93), treatment extends to 16 weeks with addition of RBV to optimize chances of attaining an SVR.[7]

Box 9.1 HCV Genotype 1a Treatment-Naïve Noncirrhotic 12 Weeks (Recommended)

Elbasvir (50 mg)/Grazoprevir (100 mg) (*No NS5A RAVs detected)
Ledipasvir (90 mg)/Sofosbuvir (400 mg)
Paritaprevir (150 mg)/Ritonavir (100 mg)/Ombitasvir (25 mg) plus twice-daily dosed Dasabuvir (250 mg) with weight-based ribavirin
Simeprevir (150 mg) + Sofosbuvir (400 mg)
Sofosbuvir (400 mg)/Velpatasvir (100 mg)
Daclatasvir (60 mg*) + Sofosbuvir (400 mg)
Glecaprevir (300 mg)/Pibrentasvir (120 mg)

> **Box 9.2 HCV Genotype 1 Treatment Failure to PEG-IFN/Ribavirin**
>
> Elbasvir (50 mg)/Grazoprevir (100 mg) (*No NS5A RAVs detected)
> Ledipasvir (90 mg)/Sofosbuvir (400 mg)
> Paritaprevir (150 mg)/Ritonavir (100 mg)/Ombitasvir (25 mg) plus twice-daily dosed Dasabuvir (250 mg) with weight-based ribavirin
> Simeprevir (150 mg) + Sofosbuvir (400 mg)
> Sofosbuvir (400 mg)/Velpatasvir (100 mg)
> Daclatasvir (60 mg*) + Sofosbuvir (400 mg)
> Glecaprevir (300 mg)/Pibrentasvir (120 mg)

Treatment-Naïve or Experienced (PEG-IFN) Compensated Cirrhosis GT1

There are also multiple therapeutic alternatives in HCV patients with cirrhosis (Boxes 9.3, 9.4, and 9.5). In GT1 patients, available regimens include LDV/SOF +/− RBV, PRoD +/− RBV, elbasvir/grazoprevir +/− RBV, SOF/VEL. SOF/SIM +/− RBV, GLE/PIB and SOF/DAC. For example, the ION-1 trial demonstrated SVR12 rates greater than 95% using a fixed-dose combination of LDV/SOF.[8] The ASTRAL-1 trial revealed SVR rates of greater than 99% in GT1 cirrhotic patients with SOF/VEL.[9]

More recently, the EXPEDITION-1 study highlighted the success of a pangenotypic regimen of GLE/PIB without RBV for 12 weeks for HCV GT1 patients (also GT2, 4, 5, or 6) and compensated cirrhosis.[10] SVR rates of 99% were observed.

> **Box 9.3 HCV Genotype 1 Treatment Failure to PEG-IFN/Ribavirin in Compensated Cirrhosis**
>
> Elbasvir (50 mg)/Grazoprevir (100 mg) (*No NS5A RAVs detected)
> Sofosbuvir (400 mg)/Velpatasvir (100 mg)
> Glecaprevir (300 mg)/Pibrentasvir (120 mg)

> **Box 9.4 HCV Genotype 1a Treatment-Naïve Compensated Cirrhosis 12 Weeks (Recommended)**
>
> Elbasvir (50 mg)/Grazoprevir (100 mg) (*No NS5A RAVs detected)
> Ledipasvir (90 mg)/Sofosbuvir (400 mg)
> Sofosbuvir (400 mg)/Velpatasvir (100 mg)
> Glecaprevir (300 mg)/Pibrentasvir (120 mg)

> **Box 9.5 HCV Genotype 1b Treatment-Naïve Compensated Cirrhosis 12 Weeks (Recommended)**
>
> Elbasvir (50 mg)/Grazoprevir (100 mg) (*No NS5A RAVs detected)
> Ledipasvir (90 mg)/Sofosbuvir (400 mg)
> Paritaprevir (150 mg)/Ritonavir (100 mg)/Ombitasvir (25 mg) plus twice-daily dosed dasabuvir (250 mg)
> Sofosbuvir (400 mg)/Velpatasvir (100 mg)
> Glecaprevir (300 mg)/Pibrentasvir (120 mg)

Treatment Failure to PEG-IFN + PI for GT1

Several regimens are available for these patients as well (Box 9.6). These include SOF/VEL, LDV/SOF for 12–24 weeks (depending on cirrhosis status), elbasvir/grazoprevir + RBV or GLE/PIB.

Therapies for DAA Failures GT1

The vast majority of patients treated with DAA regimens achieve SVR. However, a small percentage does not. The vast majority of patients who fail therapy develop RASs that not only contribute to failure of the initial DAA regimen, but may also adversely impact response rates with subsequent therapies. Patients who have previously been exposed to regimens with an NS5A inhibitor often develop long-lasting, problematic RASs that have cross-resistance to other NS5A inhibitors.

Fortunately, there are newly approved therapies that are well-tolerated and have high efficacy in patients who have failed DAAs.

The aforementioned combination of SOF/VEL has proved to be a successful regimen with pan-genotypic coverage. As well, the addition of VOX was successful in treatment of DAA failures in the POLARIS-1 (NS5a inhibitor-experienced) and POLARIS-4 (DAA-experienced, no NS5A exposure) studies in which SVR12 was achieved in 96% and 97%, respectively.[11–13] SOF/VEL/VOX was recently approved for patients who were previously exposed to an NS5A inhibitor and failed (any genotype). It also was approved for patients who were treated with DAAs but not an NS5A inhibitor in patients with GT1a (and GT3). SOF/VEL alone was highly and equally effective in those patients with GT1b (and GT2, 4, 5, 6).[14] In addition, GLE/PIB has been approved for treatment of patients who have failed therapy with an NS5A inhibitor or PI inhibitor (but who were not exposed to both classes). The MAGELLAN-1 study demonstrated success in GT1 patients who previously failed a prior DAA with SVR rates of 95%.[15] Another pan-genotypic combination including grazoprevir, the new NS5A inhibitor ruzasvir, and the new NS5B PI uprifosbuvir has also not only shown high SVR12 rates in general HCV patient populations, but also in patients who previously failed ledipasvir-sofosbuvir and elbasvir/grazoprevir, with SVR8 in 98% in the group that received RBV for 16 weeks and 100% in the group that did not receive RBV for 24 weeks.[16-17] Unfortunately, development of this regimen was recently halted.

Box 9.6 HCV Genotype 1 Treatment Failure to Protease Inhibitors

Ledipasvir/Sofosbuvir (× 12 weeks if noncirrhotic, 24 weeks if cirrhotic)
Sofosbuvir/Velpatasvir × 12 weeks
Elbasvir/Grazoprevir + Ribavirin × 12 weeks (*check RAS)
Daclatasvir/Sofosbuvir +/− Ribavrin (12 weeks if noncirrhotic, 24 weeks with ribavirin if cirrhotic)
Sofosbuvir/Velpatasvir/Voxilaprevir × 12 weeks
Glecaprevir (300 mg)/Pibrentasvir (120 mg) × 12–16 weeks

> **Box 9.7 Genotype 4 Treatment-Naïve Noncirrhotic and Compensated Cirrhosis 12 Weeks**
>
> Paritaprevir (150 mg)/Ritonavir (100 mg)/Ombitasvir (25 mg) with weight-based ribavirin (FDC)
> Ledipasvir (90 mg)/Sofosbuvir (400 mg)
> Elbasvir (50 mg)/Grazoprevir (100 mg)
> Sofosbuvir (400 mg)/Velpatasvir (100 mg)
> Sofosbuvir/Velpatasvir/Voxilaprevir × 12 weeks
> Glecaprevir (300 mg)/Pibrentasvir (120 mg) × 12–16 weeks

Current Treatment Options for GT4

Several options exist for treatment of GT4, with similar efficacy (Box 9.7). These include LDV/SOF SOF/VEL, SOF/VEL/VOX, elbasvir-grazoprevir, GLE/PIB, and PRO + RBV. The selection of a treatment option primarily is dependent upon potential for drug interactions, availability, and cost.

Current Treatment Options for GT5/6

LDV/SOF, SOF/VEL, SOF/VEL/VOX, and GLE/PIB are highly effective and approved for therapy of patients with HCV GT5 or 6 (Box 9.8).

Conclusion

Patients infected with HCV GT1, 4–6 have evolved from a difficult to treat population in the interferon era to an easier to treat population now with a myriad of options that yield superior SVR rates and excellent tolerability. Many therapeutic options are available for most patient types. The choice of an agent commonly depends upon availability. However, certain regimens are optimal in patients with renal insufficiency and others in decompensated liver disease (the PI class is contraindicated). RBV-free regimens are ideal if available. If not, potential contraindications to RBV must be considered, and serum hemoglobin must be monitored. Vigilance regarding DDIs is important, and providers must be aware of concomitant medications that are possible contraindications to a particular regimen. Whether or not a patient has cirrhosis, if they have failed therapy in the past, the HCV GT1 subtype or the presence of baseline NS5A RASs may dictate which regimen is used or how a particular

> **Box 9.8 HCV Genotype 5/6 Treatment-Naïve Noncirrhotic and Compensated Cirrhosis 12 Weeks (Recommended)**
>
> Sofosbuvir (400 mg)/Velpatasvir (100 mg)
> Ledipasvir (90 mg)/Sofosbuvir (400 mg)
> Sofosbuvir/Velpatasvir/Voxilaprevir × 12 weeks
> Glecaprevir (300 mg)/Pibrentasvir (120 mg) × 12–16 weeks

> **Box 9.9 New HCV DAA Therapies Expected to be Approved**
>
> Grazoprevir (GZR) + Ruzasvir (RZV) + MK-3682
> Ruzasvir (RZV) + MK-3682

regimen is used (length of therapy or whether or not RBV is recommended). Patients who have failed a DAA regimen currently have new options; (Box 9.9). Although the field continues to evolve rapidly, the AASLD/IDSA guidance document should be consulted for updated recommendations for therapy of patients with HCV.

References

1. Asselah T, Marcellin P. Optimal IFN-free therapy in treatment-naive patients with HCV genotype 1 infection. *Liver Int*. 2015;35(Suppl 1):56–64.

2. Poynard T, Marcellin P, Lee SS, et al. Randomised trial of interferon alpha2b plus ribavirin for 48 weeks or for 24 weeks versus interferon alpha2b plus placebo for 48 weeks for treatment of chronic infection with hepatitis C virus. International Hepatitis Interventional Therapy Group (IHIT). *Lancet*. 1998;352(9138):1426–1432.

3. Lai MY, Kao JH, Yang PM, et al. Long-term efficacy of ribavirin plus interferon alfa in the treatment of chronic hepatitis C. *Gastroenterology*. 1996;111(5):1307–1312.

4. McHutchison JG, Everson GT, Gordon SC, et al. Telaprevir with peginterferon and ribavirin for chronic HCV genotype 1 infection. *N Engl J Med*. 2009;360(18):1827–1838.

5. Hayashi N, Okanoue T, Tsubouchi H, Toyota J, Chayama K, Kumada H. Efficacy and safety of telaprevir: a new protease inhibitor, for difficult-to-treat patients with genotype 1 chronic hepatitis C. *J Viral Hepat*. 2012;19(2):e134–e142.

6. Sherman KE, Flamm SL, Afdhal NH, et al. Response-guided telaprevir combination treatment for hepatitis C virus infection. *N Engl J Med*. 2011;365(11):1014–1024.

7. Zeuzem S, Ghalib R, Reddy KR, et al. Grazoprevir-Elbasvir combination therapy for treatment-naive cirrhotic and noncirrhotic patients with chronic hepatitis C virus genotype 1, 4, or 6 infection: a randomized trial. *Ann Intern Med*. 2015;163(1):1–13.

8. Afdhal N, Zeuzem S, Kwo P, et al. Ledipasvir and sofosbuvir for untreated HCV genotype 1 infection. *N Engl J Med*. 2014;370(20):1889–1898.

9. Feld JJ, Jacobson IM, Hezode C, et al. Sofosbuvir and Velpatasvir for HCV genotype 1, 2, 4, 5, and 6 infection. *N Engl J Med*. 2015;373(27):2599–2607.

10. Forns X, Lee S, Valdes J, et al. EXPEDITION-1: efficacy and safety of Glecaprevir/Pibrentasvir in adults with chronic hepatitis C virus genotype 1, 2, 4, 5 or 6 infection and compensated cirrhosis. Presented at The International Liver Congress (ILC) in Amsterdam, The Netherlands, April 19–23, 2017.

11. Gane E, Kowdley KV, Pound D, et al. Efficacy of Sofosbuvir, Velpatasvir, and GS-9857 in patients with hepatitis C virus genotype 2, 3, 4, or 6 infections in an open-label, phase 2 trial. *Gastroenterology*. 2016; 151(5):902–909.

12. Rodriguez-Torres M, Glass S, Hill J, et al. GS-9857 in patients with chronic hepatitis C virus genotype 1-4 infection: a randomized, double-blind, dose-ranging phase 1 study. *J Viral Hepat*. 2016;23(8):614–622.

13. Lawitz E, Reau N, Hinestrosa F, et al. Efficacy of Sofosbuvir, Velpatasvir, and GS-9857 in patients with genotype 1 hepatitis C virus infection in an open-label, phase 2 trial. *Gastroenterology*. 2016; 151(5):893–901.
14. Bourlière M, Gordon SC, Flamm SL, et al. Sofosbuvir, velpatasvir, and voxilaprevir for previously treated HCV infection. *N Engl J Med*. 2017;376(22):2134–2146.
15. Gane E, Poordad F, Wang S, et al. High efficacy of ABT-493 and ABT-530 treatment in patients with HCV genotype 1 or 3 infection and compensated cirrhosis. *Gastroenterology*. 2016;151(4):651–659.e1.
16. Wedemeyer H, Wyles D, Reddy R, et al. Safety and efficacy of the fixed-dose combination regimen of MK- 3682/grazoprevir/ruzasvir in cirrhotic or non-cirrhotic patients with chronic HCV GT1 infection who previously failed a direct- acting antiviral regimen (C-SURGE). EASL International Liver Congress. Amsterdam, April 19–23, 2017. Abstract PS-159
17. Lawitz E, Yoshida EM, Buti M, et al. Safety and efficacy of the fixed-dose combination regimen of MK-3682/Grazoprevir/MK-8408 (Ruzasvir) with or without Ribavirin in non-cirrhotic or cirrhotic patients with chronic HCV GT1, 2 or 3 infection (Part B of C-CREST-1 & -2). *Lancet Gastroenterology and Hepatology*. 2017;2(11): 814–823.

Chapter 10

Treatment of Hepatitis C Genotypes 2 and 3

Deepak Venkat and Stanley Martin Cohen

Introduction

To date, six major genotypes of chronic hepatitis C virus (HCV) have been identified. Worldwide, genotype 1 (GT1) accounts for the most infections (83.4 million), followed by genotype 3 (GT3; 54.3 million), and then genotype 2 (GT2; 16.5 million).[1] In the United States, GT1 is the most common, accounting for more than 70% of infections, while GT2 and GT3 account for about 15% and 10% of infections, respectively.[2]

HCV is associated with a 75–85% likelihood of developing a chronic infection. Of those, 20–25% will develop cirrhosis. Among those who develop cirrhosis, 20% will develop hepatocellular carcinoma (HCC). Extrahepatic manifestations including cryoglobulinemia, membranoproliferative glomerulonephritis, and dermatologic manifestations can also occur with HCV. Thus, treatment for HCV is important in order to eradicate the virus, which may prevent—or at least slow—disease progression and the development of associated complications.

Traditionally, GT2 and GT3 were considered together because of similar expected sustained virologic response (SVR) rates in the era of treatment with pegylated-interferon (PEG-IFN) and ribavirin (RBV)-based therapy. However, in the era of direct-acting antivirals (DAAs) for the treatment of HCV, it has become clear that GT2 is more responsive than GT3, thus meriting consideration of these genotypes in separate categories. In fact, while SVR rates for genotypes 1 and 2 are well in excess of 90% in most DAA studies, GT3 response rates, especially in cirrhotic prior nonresponders, are often substantially lower. This may be attributable to accelerated fibrosis progression and development of significant steatosis in GT3 patients relative to other genotypes.[3–4] Comparatively, GT2 appears to be the least fibrogenic, perhaps accounting for increased responsiveness to therapy.

This chapter will focus on treatment of HCV genotypes 2 and 3. Significant guidance for these treatment recommendations comes from the American Association for the Study of Liver Diseases and the Infectious Disease Society of America (AASLD-IDSA) guidance document in the United States.[5] We have also included some input from the European Association for the Study of Liver (EASL) guidelines in the European Union.[6] Of note, the AASLD-IDSA guidance document has been updated since the approval of glecaprevir and pibrentasvir, while the EASL guidelines have not.

Goals of Treatment

The ultimate goal of all HCV treatment regimens is the achievement of SVR, defined as an undetectable HCV RNA level measured by highly sensitive polymerase chain reaction (PCR) after the end of treatment. SVR essentially equates to a "cure" of HCV and appears to be more than 99% durable.[7] SVR leads to improved liver histology, delayed disease progression, and decreased complications of chronic HCV infection.[8] A VA study demonstrated that SVR was associated with a 30–49% reduction in all-cause mortality in patients with HCV.[9]

Previous regimens used SVR24 (HCV RNA negative 24 weeks after stopping therapy) as their endpoint. More recently, SVR12 (HCV RNA negative 12 weeks after stopping treatment) has been considered the standard of care for defining SVR.[10] This definition has also been accepted by the US Food and Drug Administration (FDA) in their evaluation of HCV studies.

Pretreatment Testing

Pretreatment testing is addressed in Chapter 4. The pretreatment testing for HCV GT2 is the same as the other genotypes.

However, unique to GT3 is the fact that outcomes of DAA therapy for HCV GT3 can be affected by the presence of resistance-associated substitutions (RAS), especially the Y93H mutation. Because of this, DAA regimens vary depending on the presence or absence of Y93H. The AASLD-IDSA guidance document and the EASL guidelines recommend RAS testing in certain populations of HCV GT3 patients as outlined below and in the tables.[6]

Treatment for HCV Genotypes 2 and 3

The major predictors of response to the treatment of HCV with DAAs are prior treatment experience, degree of fibrosis, and the presence of RAS (in GT3 patients). Thus, we have broken down treatment recommendations accordingly with a focus on major societal recommendations from the AASLD-IDSA and EASL. Please note that the AASLD-IDSA guidance document is web-based and is constantly being updated. We strongly recommend that the reader refer to this document at hcvguidelines.org to get the most updated information because the data and recommendations change frequently.

Older Treatment Regimens for Genotypes 2 and 3

Prior to the availability of DAA therapy, the standard of care for genotypes 2 and 3 was 24 weeks of weekly PEG-IFN injections and a fixed oral dose of 800 mg of RBV daily. Expected overall SVR rates for GT2 and GT3 patients treated with this regimen were 76–82%.[11,12] However, patients with GT3 with advanced fibrosis or cirrhosis remained poorly responsive, with expected SVR rates of less than 50%, even with extension of therapy to 48 weeks.[13]

In addition to suboptimal SVR rates, patients treated with PEG-IFN and RBV experienced a variety of side effects and toxicities. Because of this, patients had to be willing to consider the risks and benefits of such therapies. Particular attention needed to be paid to baseline characteristics and contraindications to therapy. In addition, caution needed to be exercised in patients with advanced liver disease, often leading to the exclusion of patients with Child's B and C cirrhosis from treatment with PEG-IFN–based therapy. Because of the anticipated hematologic effects, patients with advanced cardiac comorbidities were also considered high risk for or excluded from therapy. Absolute contraindications to PEG-IFN and RBV therapy included severe mental illness, autoimmune disease, untreated thyroid disease, pregnancy, severe uncontrolled cardiopulmonary comorbidities (congestive heart failure, chronic obstructive pulmonary disease, coronary artery disease), and known hypersensitivity to the medications.

Because RBV still has a role in some of the treatment regimens for HCV genotypes 2 and 3, clinicians still need to be aware of the potential side effects of this medication. The main issues include hemolytic anemia, rash, and teratogenicity. Due to renal clearance of this medication, the hemolytic anemia may be more pronounced in patients with renal insufficiency. Closer monitoring of blood counts and/or adjustment in RBV dosing may be necessary in such patients.

Until recently, the combination of PEG-IFN and low-dose RBV was recommended by the guidelines for HCV GT2 and GT3 patients with renal failure (CrCl <30 or dialysis). However, with the late 2017 approval of glecaprevir (a protease inhibitor) and pibrentasvir (an NS5A inhibitor), including in patients with renal failure, PEG-IFN and RBV are no longer a recommended regimen for such patients.

Currently Available DAA Agents for HCV Genotypes 2 and 3

Considerable research over the past few years has led to the development of newer, more effective and less toxic agents for HCV. Sofosbuvir (Sovaldi®) is an HCV DAA.[14] It is a nucleotide analogue inhibitor of the NS5B polymerase enzyme of the HCV genome. It is a fixed-dose oral pill, taken once daily, with pan-genomic activity against HCV genotypes 1–6 with a high barrier to resistance. Because of these attributes, it has become the backbone of several FDA-approved treatment regimens for all genotypes of HCV.

In clinical trials, the most common side effects to sofosbuvir itself were fatigue and headache (≥20%). However, another consideration in its use is the potential for drug–drug interactions. Some of these are outlined in Table 10.1.[14] As noted in the table, such interactions can occur with a variety of medications and herbal products. Coadministration with such agents is not recommended. In addition, sofosbuvir has not been studied extensively in patients with creatinine clearance of less than 30, patients with end-stage renal disease, and those on dialysis, so its use cannot be recommended in these populations.

Table 10.1 Drugs with significant interactions with sofosbuvir

Drug Class	Clinical Effect
ANTIARRHYTHMICS: Amiodarone	Can cause significant bradycardia. Coadministration is not recommended.
ANTICONVULSANTS: Carbamazepine Phenytoin Phenobarbital Oxcarbazepine	Coadministration of anticonvulsants reduces concentration of sofosbuvir. Coadministration is not recommended
ANTIMYCOBACTERIALS: Rifabutin Rifampin Rifapentine	Coadministration of antimycobacterial reduces concentration of sofosbuvir. Coadministration is not recommended
HERBAL SUPPLEMENTS: St. John's Wort	Coadministration of St. John's Wort reduces concentration of sofosbuvir. Coadministration is not recommended.
HIV PROTEASE INHIBITORS: Tipranavir/Ritonavir	Coadministration of HIV protease inhibitors Tipranavir/Ritonavir reduces concentration of sofosbuvir. Coadministration is not recommended.

Note: The following medications had no significant drug interactions in clinical trials: cyclosporine, tacrolimus, tenofovir, darunavir/ritonavir, efavirenz, emtricitabine, methadone, oral contraceptives, raltegrevir, rilpivirine.

Velpatasvir is an NS5A inhibitor that is used in combination with sofosbuvir as a single-tablet regimen (Epclusa® when combined with sofosbuvir) to treat HCV genotypes 2 and 3.[15] The most commonly observed adverse events with the combination drug were headache, fatigue, and nausea. Because sofosbuvir is the backbone of sofosbuvir/velpatasvir combination therapy, all of the same potential drug–drug interactions are present with the combination drug as outlined in Table 10.1. The combination should not be coadministered with oxcarbazepine, phenobarbital, phenytoin, rifabutin, rifapentine, and tipranavir/ritonavir due to possibly decreased concentrations of sofosbuvir and/or velpatasvir. Also, coadministration of sofosbuvir/velpatasvir is not recommended with proton pump inhibitors (PPI) or efavirenz due to decreased concentrations of velpatasvir. If it is medically necessary to coadminister with a PPI, sofosbuvir/velpatasvir should be administered with food and taken 4 hours before the equivalent of omeprazole 20 mg daily. Also, sofosbuvir/velpatasvir should not be coadministered with topotecan due to possibly increased concentrations of topotecan.[15]

Sofosbuvir/velpatasvir does not require dose adjustments in geriatric patients, cirrhotic patients, or patients with mild to moderate renal impairment. However, safety and efficacy of the combination has not been established in pediatric patients or patients with severe renal impairment (GFR <30 mL/min) and can thus not be recommended in these populations.

Daclatasvir (Daklinza®) is another NS5A inhibitor that is used in combination with sofosbuvir for the treatment of HCV genotypes 2 and 3.[16] Daclatasvir is generally prescribed as a 60 mg tablet daily. To allow for possible dosage adjustments of this medication (see information on possible drug interactions in the following section), Daclatasvir is available in 30 mg, 60 mg, and 90 mg tablets. The most common adverse events are nausea, fatigue, and headache. Because sofosbuvir is the backbone of sofosbuvir and daclatasvir therapy, all of the same potential drug–drug interactions are present with the combination treatment as outlined in Table 10.1. In addition, daclatasvir is a substrate of cytochrome P3A (CYP3A). Moderate or strong inducers of CYP3A can decrease daclatasvir levels, which may necessitate increasing the dosage of daclatasvir. Strong inducers of CYP3A such as phenytoin, carbamazepine, rifampin, and St. John's wort are contraindicated with daclatasvir. On the other hand, strong inhibitors such as clarithromycin, ketoconazole, and ritonavir may increase daclatasvir levels, which may necessitate decreasing the dosage of daclatasvir. In addition, daclatasvir is an inhibitor of P-gp, OATP 1B1 and 1B3, and breast cancer receptor protein (BCRP). As such, daclatasvir may increase levels of substrates, actively increasing their potential toxicity.

Daclatasvir does not require dose adjustments in patients with mild, moderate, or severe hepatic impairment (Child's A, B, or C patients) or with any level of renal impairment. However, because it is used with sofosbuvir, the combination is not recommended in patients with severe renal impairment (GFR <30 mL/min).

Glecaprevir (a protease inhibitor) used in combination with pibrentasvir (an NS5A inhibitor) marketed in combination as Mavyret® was approved for HCV treatment in late 2017. It is prescribed as 3 tablets daily. Each tablet contains 100 mg of glecaprevir and 40 mg of pibrentasvir. This is a pangenotypic medication that is approved for treating HCV GT2 and GT3. The most commonly observed adverse events include headache, fatigue, and nausea. Significant decreases in therapeutic effect can be seen with the combination of glecaprevir/pibrentasvir and carbamazepine or efavirenz or St. John's wort, and these mediations should not be combined with this HCV regimen. In addition, this regimen should not be used with atazanavir or rifampin.

Glecaprevir/pibrentasvir should not be used in patients with severe hepatic impairment (Child's class C patients). It does not require any dose adjustments for any level of renal impairment.

First-Generation DAA Treatment Regimen for HCV GT 2

The first interferon-free, DAA regimen for HCV GT2 was sofosbuvir and RBV for 12 weeks, based on the combined data from several trials.[17–20]

For treatment-naïve GT2 patients in the FISSION trial, 12 weeks of oral sofosbuvir and weight-based RBV achieved an SVR of 97% in treatment-naïve patients compared to 78% who received 24 weeks of PEG-IFN and RBV.[17] Not unexpectedly, the patients in the PEG-IFN/ribavirin arm suffered significantly more and worse side effects compared to the oral sofosbuvir

+ RBV regimen. In the POSITRON trial, 12 weeks of oral sofosbuvir and weight-based RBV achieved an SVR12 in 93% of treatment-naïve patients, regardless of the presence or absence of cirrhosis/advanced fibrosis.[18] In the VALENCE trial, 12 weeks of oral sofosbuvir and weight-based RBV achieved an SVR in 97% of treatment-naïve noncirrhotic patients and 100% of cirrhotic patients.[19]

For interferon- and RBV-experienced GT2 patients, in the FUSION trial, treatment-experienced patients were randomized to receive 12 or 16 weeks of sofosbuvir + weight-based RBV[20]; 86% of treatment-experienced patients receiving 12 weeks of therapy had SVR versus 94% in the 16-week arm. In patients without cirrhosis, 96% in the 12-week arm and 100% in the 16-week arm achieved an SVR12. However, in patients with cirrhosis, only 60% of patients in the 12-week arm versus 78% in the 16-week arm achieved an SVR12. In the VALENCE study, 12 weeks of sofosbuvir + weight-based RBV achieved an overall 90% SVR in treatment-experienced GT2 HCV patients.[19] Of that group, 91% of noncirrhotic patients achieved an SVR12 versus 88% of cirrhotic patients.

Due to the side effects associated with RBV as well as the development of newer DAA regimens which did not require the use of RBV, the guidelines changed in 2016. *Sofosbuvir + RBV is no longer included in the AASLD-IDSA guidance document and is listed as "suboptimal" in the latest EASL guidelines.*[5,6]

Currently Recommended DAA Treatment Regimens for HCV GT 2

Table 10.2 lists the currently recommended DAA treatment regimens for HCV GT2. These are based on the AASLD-IDSA guidance document and EASL guidelines.[5,6]

Genotype 2, Treatment-Naïve

The current treatment regimens for the treatment-naïve GT2 patients are outlined in Table 10.2. The sofosbuvir/velpatasvir regimen is a recommended regimen per the AASLD-IDSA and a first-line regimen per the EASL guidelines; it is given for 12 weeks whether or not the patient has cirrhosis. The glecaprevir/pibrentasvir regimen is a recommended regimen per the AASLD-IDSA guidance document; it is given for 8 weeks in those without cirrhosis and for 12 weeks in those with compensated cirrhosis. The sofosbuvir and daclatasvir regimen (an alternative regimen per AASLD-IDSA and a first-line regimen per EASL) varies in length based on the presence or absence of cirrhosis.

The combination of sofosbuvir/velpatasvir was studied for HCV GT2 patients in the ASTRAL 1 and ASTRAL 2 trials.[21,22] These studies included treatment-naïve and treatment-experienced (IFN and RBV) patients with or without compensated cirrhosis. ASTRAL 1 was a placebo-controlled trial. The SVR was 100% (104/104) in the sofosbuvir/velpatasvir group. ASTRAL 2 compared sofosbuvir/velpatasvir to the standard of care (at the time) of sofosbuvir and RBV. The SVR was 99% (133/134) in the sofosbuvir/velpatasvir group compared to 94% in the sofosbuvir + RBV group. Overall, only

Table 10.2 Treatment of HCV genotype 2

Clinical Features	AASLD-IDSA (Rating: Class and Level)	EASL (Grade: Quality and Recommendation)	SVR Rates[a]
Treatment-naïve without cirrhosis	• Glecaprevir 300 mg/Pibrentasvir 120 mg daily × 8 weeks (recommended regimen) (I, A) • Sofosbuvir 400 mg/Velpatasvir 100 mg daily × 12 weeks (recommended regimen) (I, A) • Sofosbuvir 400 mg and Daclatasvir 60 mg daily × 12 weeks (alternative regimen) (IIa, B)	• Sofosbuvir 400 mg/Velpatasvir 100 mg daily × 12 weeks (first-line option) (A1) • Sofosbuvir 400 mg and Daclatasvir 60 mg daily × 12 weeks (first-line option) (B1)	• 98–100% (SURVEYOR-2 and EXPEDITION-1) • 99–100% (ASTRAL 1 and 2) • 100% (ALLY 2) • 92% (AI444040)
Treatment-naïve with compensated cirrhosis	• Glecaprevir 300 mg/Pibrentasvir 120 mg daily × 12 weeks (recommended regimen) (I, B) • Sofosbuvir 400 mg/Velpatasvir 100 mg daily × 12 weeks (recommended regimen) (I, A) • Sofosbuvir 400 mg and Daclatasvir 60 mg daily × 16–24 weeks (alternative regimen) (IIa, B)	• Sofosbuvir 400 mg/Velpatasvir 100 mg daily × 12 weeks (first-line option) (A1) • Sofosbuvir 400 mg and Daclatasvir 60 mg daily × 12 weeks (first-line option per EASL) (B1)	• 99% (EXPEDITION-1) • 99–100% (ASTRAL 1 and 2) • 100% (ALLY 2)
Treatment-experienced to IFN and RBV without cirrhosis	• Glecaprevir 300 mg/Pibrentasvir 120 mg daily × 8 weeks (recommended regimen) (I, A) • Sofosbuvir 400 mg/Velpatasvir 100 mg daily × 12 weeks (recommended regimen) (I, A) • Sofosbuvir 400 mg and Daclatasvir 60 mg daily × 12 weeks (alternative regimen) (IIa, B)	• Sofosbuvir 400 mg/Velpatasvir 100 mg daily × 12 weeks (first-line option) (A1) • Sofosbuvir 400 mg and Daclatasvir 60 mg daily × 12 weeks (first-line option) (B1)	• 98% (SURVEYOR-2) • 99–100% (ASTRAL 1 and 2)
Treatment-experienced to IFN and RBV with compensated cirrhosis	• Glecaprevir 300 mg/Pibrentasvir 120 mg daily × 12 weeks (recommended regimen) (I, B) • Sofosbuvir 400 mg/Velpatasvir 100 mg daily × 12 weeks (recommended regimen) (I, A) • Sofosbuvir 400 mg and Daclatasvir 60 mg daily × 16–24 weeks (alternative regimen) (IIa, B)	• Sofosbuvir 400 mg/Velpatasvir 100 mg daily × 12 weeks (first-line option) (A1) • Sofosbuvir 400 mg and Daclatasvir 60 mg daily × 12 weeks (first-line option) (B1)	• 100% (EXPEDITION-1) • 99–100% (ASTRAL 1 and 2)

(continued)

Table 10-2 Continued

Clinical Features	AASLD-IDSA (Rating: Class and Level)	EASL (Grade: Quality and Recommendation)	SVR Rates[a]
Treatment-experienced to Sofosbuvir and RBV with or without compensated cirrhosis	• Glecaprevir 300 mg/Pibrentasvir 120 mg daily + RBV × 12 weeks (recommended regimen) (IIb, B) • Sofosbuvir 400 mg/Velpatasvir 100 mg daily + RBV × 12 weeks (recommended regimen) (IIa, C)	• Sofosbuvir 400 mg/Velpatasvir 100 mg daily + RBV × 12 weeks (recommended regimen if F0–F2) (B2) • Sofosbuvir 400 mg/Velpatasvir 100 mg daily + RBV × 24 weeks (recommended regimen if F3–F4) (B2) • Sofosbuvir 400 mg and Daclatasvir 60 mg daily + RBV × 12 weeks (recommended regimen if F0–F2) (B2) • Sofosbuvir 400 mg and Daclatasvir 60 mg daily + RBV × 24 weeks (recommended regimen if F3–F4) (B2)	• 99-100% (ENDURANCE-2 and EXPEDITION-1) • 97% (POLARIS-4)
Decompensated cirrhosis (Child's class B or C)	• Sofosbuvir 400 mg/Velpatasvir 100 mg daily + RBV × 12 weeks (recommended regimen) (I, A) • Sofosbuvir 400 mg/Velpatasvir 100 mg daily × 24 weeks (if unable to take RBV) (recommended regimen) (I, A) • Sofosbuvir 400 mg and Daclatasvir 60 mg daily + RBV × 12 weeks (recommended regimen) (II, B) • Sofosbuvir 400 mg and Daclatasvir 60 mg daily × 24 weeks (if unable to take RBV) (recommended regimen) (II, C)	• Sofosbuvir 400 mg/Velpatasvir 100 mg daily + RBV × 12 weeks (recommended regimen) (B1) • Sofosbuvir 400 mg/Velpatasvir 100 mg daily × 24 weeks (recommended regimen, if unable to tolerate RBV) (B1) • Sofosbuvir 400 mg and Daclatasvir 60 mg daily + RBV × 12 weeks (recommended regimen) (B1) • Sofosbuvir 400 mg and Daclatasvir 60 mg daily × 24 weeks (recommended regimen, if unable to tolerate RBV) (B1)	• 100% (ASTRAL 4) • 80% (ALLY 1)

[a] Sustained virologic response (SVR) rates from selected studies. Some are limited by small numbers. These are not meant to be head-to-head comparisons. See the text for more details.

0.2% of patients discontinued their sofosbuvir/velpatasvir due to adverse events across the entire ASTRAL program.

The combination of glecaprevir/pibrentasvir was studied for HCV GT2 patients in the SURVEYOR-2 and EXPEDITION-1 trials.[23,24] In SURVEYOR-2, noncirrhotic treatment-naïve patients (and those who had failed prior interferon and ribavirin), the SVR was 98% (193/197) with an 8-week course of therapy. In EXPEDITION-1, treatment-naïve patients (and those who had failed prior interferon and ribavirin) with compensated cirrhosis had an SVR of 100% (31/31). Overall, only 0.1% of patients discontinued their glecaprevir/pibrentasvir due to adverse events across the entire registration trial program.

The combination of sofosbuvir and daclatasvir also reveals excellent SVR rates in treatment-naïve GT2 patients in various studies.[25,26] In the ALLY 2 study, which allowed cirrhotic patients, a 100% (17/17) SVR rate was seen.[25] In the AI444040 study, Sulkowski et al. randomized GT2 naïve patients to various 24-week regimens of sofosbuvir and daclatasvir with and without RBV.[26] They had a 92% SVR rate. As note in Table 10.2, there are some differences between the EASL and AASLD-IDSA guidelines on length of therapy based on the presence or absence of compensated cirrhosis. For treatment-naïve GT2 patients with compensated cirrhosis, the AASLD-IDSA guidance document recommends prolonging therapy with this regimen to 16–24 weeks, while the EASL guidelines recommend a 12-week course of therapy.

Genotype 2, Treatment-Experienced

The guidelines for these patients vary based on whether patients had been previous nonresponders to IFN-based therapy or DAA-based regimens as outlined in Table 10.2.

The latest guidelines now support the use of glecaprevir/pibrentasvir, sofosbuvir/velpatasvir or sofosbuvir and daclatasvir for the IFN-experienced GT2 patients.

As noted earlier, the SURVEYOR-2 and EXPEDITION-1 trials of glecaprevir/pibrentasvir combined treatment-naïve patients and those who had failed PEG-IFN and RBV.[23,24] The SVR rates were excellent as above, and the AASLD-IDSA guidelines suggest 8 weeks for noncirrhotic patients and 12 weeks for cirrhotic patients who are PEG-IFN- and RBV-experienced.

In the ASTRAL 2 study, 12 weeks of sofosbuvir/velpatasvir (134 total patients of whom 19 were treatment-experienced) was significantly better than 12 weeks of sofosbuvir and RBV (SVR rates of 99% and 94%, respectively).[22]

Data on the use of sofosbuvir and daclatasvir in this group are more limited. The ALLY 2 study only included two HCV GT2 treatment-experienced patients, and both achieved SVR.[25] The AASLD-IDSA guidance document considers this as an alternative regimen for 12 weeks in non-cirrhotic patients and recommends extending such therapy to 16–24 weeks in patients with compensated cirrhosis. However, the EASL guidelines consider this a first-line option for 12 weeks, with or without cirrhosis.

Given the relatively high SVR rates even with the combination of sofosbuvir and RBV, most clinicians will not see many patients who failed this previous regimen. In addition, there is little published data on such patients. Most of the guidelines in this group are based on small studies and extrapolated data. For this group, AASLD-IDSA recommends 12 weeks of sofosbuvir/velpatasvir or 12 weeks of glecaprevir/pibrentasvir. As noted in Table 10.2 the EASL guidelines look at stage of fibrosis to determine if sofosbuvir/velpatasvir and weight-based RBV or sofosbuvir and daclatasvir and weight-based RBV should be used for 12 weeks (if stage 0–2 fibrosis) or 24 weeks (if stage 3–4 fibrosis).

Finally, GT2 patients who have failed therapy with sofosbuvir/velpatasvir or sofosbuvir and daclatasvir will be extremely uncommon. Firm recommendations are not currently available for the treatment of such patients. Resistance testing may be beneficial in such patients. Longer treatment durations with the addition of RBV will likely be necessary. In addition, upcoming treatment regimens may act as rescue therapies for such patients.

Genotype 2, Decompensated Cirrhosis

The treatment recommendations for decompensated GT2 HCV patients are as outlined in Table 10.2.

In the ASTRAL 4 study, the SVR rate was 100% (although very small numbers of patients were included) for decompensated GT2 HCV cirrhotic patients treated with sofosbuvir/velpatasvir with or without RBV for 12 weeks.[27]

In the ALLY 1 study, which used sofosbuvir and daclatasvir and weight-based RBV for 12 weeks in patients with advanced cirrhosis, the number of GT2 patients (only 5 patients) was too small to make firm evidence-based recommendations[28]; 80% (4/5) of patients achieved SVR in this group.

Protease inhibitors are contraindicated in those with decompensated cirrhosis, and thus glecaprevir/pibrentasvir is not a recommended regimen in this group of patients.

Treatment for HCV GT 3

As noted earlier, treating GT3 is more difficult than treating GT2. The SVR rates in GT3, especially in treatment-experienced cirrhotic patients, are not as robust as those seen in other genotypes. Several factors may account for this including more significant fibrosis, steatosis, and the presence of pretreatment RAS.

First-Generation DAA Treatment Regimen for HCV GT 3

The first IFN-free DAA regimen for HCV GT3 was sofosbuvir and RBV for 24 weeks, based on the combined data from several trials.[17–20]

For GT3 patients in the FISSION trial, 12 weeks of oral sofosbuvir and weight-based RBV achieved an SVR of 56% in treatment-naïve patients compared to 63% who received 24 weeks of PEG-IFN and RBV.[17] Cirrhotic patients in this study treated with sofosbuvir and RBV for 12 weeks only had an SVR of 34%. Not unexpectedly, the patients in the PEG-IFN/ribavirin arm suffered significantly more and worse side effects compared to the oral sofosbuvir + RBV regimen. In the POSITRON trial, 12 weeks of oral sofosbuvir and weight-based RBV achieved an SVR12 in 61% of GT3 patients.[18] Cirrhotic patients only achieved SVR in 21%. In the VALENCE trial, 24 weeks of oral sofosbuvir and weight-based RBV achieved an SVR in 85% (91% in patients without cirrhosis and 68% in patients with cirrhosis).[19] Thus, longer treatment courses were recommended for HCV GT3 therapy.

Similar to GT2, *sofosbuvir and RBV is no longer included in the AASLD-IDSA guidance document and is listed as "suboptimal" in the latest EASL guidelines for the treatment of HCV GT3 patients.*[5,6]

Currently Recommended DAA Treatment Regimens for HCV GT 3

Table 10.3 lists the currently recommended DAA treatment regimens for HCV GT3. These are based on the AASLD-IDSA guidance document and EASL guidelines.[5,6] Note that testing for NS5A Y93H RAS is recommended by both sets of guidelines in many of the GT3 patients.

Genotype 3, Treatment-Naïve, Noncirrhotic

The currently recommended treatments are outlined in Table 10.3. In the ASTRAL 3 study, 12 weeks of sofosbuvir 400 mg daily/velpatasvir 100 mg daily given to 163 treatment-naïve, noncirrhotic patients with GT3 HCV resulted in a 98% SVR12.[22] In the ENDURANCE-3 study, 8 weeks of glecprevir/pibrentasvir in treatment-naïve, noncirrhotic GT3 patients resulted in a 95% SVR rate (149/157).[29] In the ALLY 3 study, 12 weeks of sofosbuvir 400 mg daily and daclatasvir 60 mg daily given to 101 treatment-naïve, noncirrhotic patients with GT3 HCV resulted in a 97% SVR12.[30]

Genotype 3, Treatment-Naïve, with Compensated Cirrhosis

The currently recommended treatments are outlined in Table 10.3.

In the ASTRAL 3 study, sofosbuvir/velpatasvir given for 12 weeks to 43 treatment-naïve, cirrhotic patients with GT3 HCV resulted in a 93% SVR12.[22] Of those with baseline Y93H RAS, 84% achieved an SVR12. Because of this, the current AASLD-IDSA guidance document and EASL guidelines recommend testing for Y93H RAS in this population and adding weight-based RBV if present.[5,6]

In the SURVEYOR-2 study, glecaprvir/pibrenatsvir given for 12 weeks to GT3 treatment-naïve patients with compensated cirrhosis resulted in an SVR12 rate of 98% (39/40).[31]

In the ALLY 3 study, sofosbuvir 400 mg and daclatasvir 60 mg given for 12 weeks to treatment-naïve, cirrhotic patients with GT3 HCV resulted in only a 58% SVR12.[32] Because of these low SVR rates with 12 weeks of therapy, the ALLY 3+ study looked at 12 versus 16 weeks of sofosbuvir and daclatasvir with the addition of RBV in treatment-naïve or treatment-experienced patients with either advanced fibrosis or cirrhosis.[33] Overall, 88% of the 12-week patients and 92% of the 16-week patients had SVR. For the patients with stage 3 fibrosis, 100% had SVR in both groups. Specifically for the cirrhotic patients, 86% overall achieved an SVR12 (83% in the 12-week group and 89% in the 16-week arm), of whom the majority were treatment-experienced. Also, in a European compassionate use program, SVR12 rates in cirrhotic patients with GT3 HCV were improved from 70% to 86% when therapy with sofosbuvir and daclatasvir was extended from 12 to 24 weeks.[33]

Table 10.3 Treatment of HCV genotype 3

Clinical Features	AASLD-IDSA[a] (Rating: Class and Level)	EASL[b] (Grade: Quality and Recommendation)	SVR Rates[c]
Treatment-naïve without cirrhosis	- Glecaprevir 300 mg/Pibrentasvir 120 mg daily × 8 weeks (recommended regimen) (I, A) - Sofosbuvir 400 mg/Velpatasvir 100 mg daily × 12 weeks (recommended regimen) (I, A) - Sofosbuvir 400 mg and Daclatasvir 60 mg daily × 12 weeks (alternative regimen) (I, A)	- Sofosbuvir 400 mg/Velpatasvir 100 mg daily × 12 weeks (first-line option) (A1) - Sofosbuvir 400 mg and Daclatasvir 60 mg daily × 12 weeks (first-line option) (B1)	- 95% (ENDURANCE-3) - 98% (ASTRAL 3) - 97% (ALLY 3)
Treatment-naïve with compensated cirrhosis	- Glecaprevir 300 mg/Pibrentasvir 120 mg daily × 12 weeks (recommended regimen) (I, A) - Sofosbuvir 400 mg/Velpatasvir 100 mg daily × 12 weeks (recommended regimen in patients without NS5A RAS Y93H) (I, A) - Sofosbuvir 400 mg/Velpatasvir 100 mg/Voxilaprevir × 12 weeks (alternative regimen if NS5A RAS Y93H present) (I, A) - Sofosbuvir 400 mg/Velpatasvir 100 mg daily + RBV × 12 weeks (recommended regimen if NS5A RAS Y93H present) (I, A) - Sofosbuvir 400 mg and Daclatasvir 60 mg daily × 24 weeks (alternative regimen in patients without RAS Y93H) (IIa, B) - Sofosbuvir 400 mg and Daclatasvir 60 mg daily + RBV × 24 weeks (alternative regimen if RAS Y93H present) (IIa, B)	- Sofosbuvir 400 mg/Velpatasvir 100 mg daily × 12 weeks (first-line option in patients without NS5A RAS Y93H) (A1) - Sofosbuvir 400 mg/Velpatasvir 100 mg daily + RBV × 12 weeks (first-line option if RAS testing not done, or if NS5A RAS Y93H present) (A1) - Sofosbuvir 400 mg/Velpatasvir 100 mg daily × 24 weeks (first-line option if unable to receive RBV) (C1) - Sofosbuvir 400 mg and Daclatasvir 60 mg daily + RBV × 24 weeks (first-line option) (C1) - Sofosbuvir 400 mg and Daclatasvir 60 mg daily × 24 weeks (first-line option if unable to tolerate RBV) (C1)	- 93% (ASTRAL 3) (Lower with Y93H) - 96% (POLARIS-3) - 86% (European compassionate use study)

Treatment-experienced to IFN and RBV without cirrhosis	- Sofosbuvir 400 mg/Velpatasvir 100 mg daily × 12 weeks (recommended regimen) in patients without RAS Y93H) (I, A) - Sofosbuvir 400 mg/Velpatasvir 100 mg daily + RBV × 12 weeks (recommended regimen if RAS Y93H present) (I, A) - Glecaprevir 300 mg/Pibrentasvir 120 mg daily × 16 weeks (alternative regimen) (IIa, B) - Sofosbuvir 400 mg and Daclatasvir 60 mg daily × 12 weeks (alternative regimen in patients without RAS Y93H) (I, A) - Sofosbuvir 400 mg and Daclatasvir 60 mg daily + RBV × 12 weeks (alternative regimen if RAS Y93H present) (I, A) - Sofosbuvir 400 mg/Velpatasvir 100 mg/Voxilaprevir 100 mg daily × 12 weeks (alternative regimen if RAS Y93H present) (IIb, B)	- Sofosbuvir 400 mg/Velpatasvir 100 mg daily × 12 weeks (first-line option in patients without RAS Y93H) (A1) - Sofosbuvir 400 mg/Velpatasvir 100 mg daily + RBV × 12 weeks (first-line option if RAS testing not done, or if RAS Y93H present) (A1) - Sofosbuvir 400 mg/Velpatasvir 100 mg daily × 24 weeks (first-line option if unable to receive RBV) (C1) - Sofosbuvir 400 mg and Daclatasvir 60 mg daily × 12 weeks (first-line option in patients without RAS Y93H) (B1) - Sofosbuvir 400 mg and Daclatasvir 60 mg daily + RBV × 12 weeks (first-line option if RAS testing not done, or if RAS Y93H present) (B1) - Sofosbuvir 400 mg and Daclatasvir 60 mg daily × 24 weeks (first-line option if unable to tolerate RBV) (C1)	- 91% (ASTRAL 3) - 96% (SURVEYOR-2) - 94% (ALLY 3)
Treatment-experienced to IFN and RBV with compensated cirrhosis	- Elbasvir 50 mg/Grazoprevir 100 mg + Sofosbuvir 400 × 12 weeks (recommended regimen) (I, B) - Sofosbuvir 400 mg/Velpatasvir 100 mg/Voxilaprevir 100 mg daily × 12 weeks (recommended regimen) (IIb, B) - Sofosbuvir 400 mg/Velpatasvir 100 mg + RBV × 12 weeks (alternative regimen) (I, B) - Glecaprevir 300 mg/Pibrentasvir 120 mg daily × 16 weeks (alternative regimen) (IIa, B)	- Sofosbuvir 400 mg/Velpatasvir 100 mg daily × 12 weeks (first-line option in patients without RAS Y93H) (A1) - Sofosbuvir 400 mg/Velpatasvir 100 mg daily with RBV × 12 weeks (first-line option if RAS testing not done, or if RAS Y93H present) (A1) - Sofosbuvir 400 mg/Velpatasvir 100 mg daily × 24 weeks (first-line option if unable to receive RBV) (C1) - Sofosbuvir 400 mg and Daclatasvir 60 mg daily + RBV × 24 weeks (first-line option) (C1) - Sofosbuvir 400 mg and Daclatasvir 60 mg daily × 24 weeks (first-line option if unable to tolerate RBV) (C1)	- 100% (C-ISLE) - 96% (SURVEYOR-2)

(continued)

Table 10-3 Continued

Clinical Features	AASLD-IDSA[a] (Rating: Class and Level)	EASL[b] (Grade: Quality and Recommendation)	SVR Rates[c]
Treatment-experienced to Sofosbuvir and RBV with or without compensated cirrhosis	• Sofosbuvir 400 mg/Velpatasvir 100 mg/Voxilaprevir 100 mg daily × 12 weeks (recommended regimen if no prior NS5A failure) (I, A) • Sofosbuvir 400 mg/Velpatasvir 100 mg/Voxilaprevir 100 mg daily + RBV × 12 weeks (recommended regimen if prior NS5A failure) (IIa, C)	• Sofosbuvir 400 mg/Velpatasvir 100 mg + RBV × 12 weeks (recommended regimen if F0–F2) (B2) • Sofosbuvir 400 mg/Velpatasvir 100 mg daily + RBV × 24 weeks (recommended regimen if F3–F4) (B2) • Sofosbuvir 400 mg and Daclatasvir 60 mg daily + RBV × 12 weeks (recommended regimen if F0–F2) (B2) • Sofosbuvir 400 mg and Daclatasvir 60 mg daily + RBV × 24 weeks (recommended regimen if F3–F4) (B2)	
Decompensated cirrhosis (Child's class B or C)	• Sofosbuvir 400 mg/Velpatasvir 100 mg daily + RBV × 12 weeks (recommended regimen) (I, A) • Sofosbuvir 400 mg/Velpatasvir 100 mg daily × 24 weeks (if unable to take RBV) (recommended regimen) (I, A) • Sofosbuvir 400 mg and Daclatasvir 60 mg daily + RBV × 12 weeks (recommended regimen) (II, B) • Sofosbuvir 400 mg and Daclatasvir 60 mg daily × 24 weeks (if unable to take RBV) (recommended regimen) (II, C)	• Sofosbuvir 400 mg/Velpatasvir 100 mg daily + RBV × 24 weeks (recommended regimen) (A1, B1) • Sofosbuvir 400 mg/Velpatasvir 100 mg daily × 24 weeks (alternative regimen if unable to tolerate RBV) (B1) • Sofosbuvir 400 mg and Daclatasvir 60 mg daily + RBV × 24 weeks (recommended regimen) (A1, B1) • Sofosbuvir 400 mg and Daclatasvir 60 mg daily × 24 weeks (alternative regimen if unable to tolerate RBV) (B1)	• 85% (ASTRAL 4) • 50% (ASTRAL 4) • 83% (ALLY 1) • 73% (European expanded access study) • 86–88% (European Compassionate Use Study) • 86–88% (European Compassionate Use Study)

[a] American Association for the Study of Liver Diseases and the Infectious Disease Society of America (AASLD-IDSA) recommends testing for NS5A RAS Y93H in treatment-experienced, non-cirrhotics and treatment-naive, cirrhotic genotype 3 patients.
[b] European Association for the Study of Liver (EASL) recommends testing for NS5A RAS Y93H in treatment-experienced, non-cirrhotics, and treatment-naïve and treatment-experienced cirrhotics who are to receive sofosbuvir/velpatasvir. EASL recommends testing for NS5A RAS Y93H in treatment-experienced, noncirrhotic patients who are to receive sofosbuvir and daclatasvir (all cirrhotic patients receive 24 weeks of sofosbuvir and daclatasvir and RBV whether they have Y93H or not).
[c] SVR rates from selected studies. Some are limited by small numbers. These are not meant to be head-to-head comparisons. See the text for more details.

The impact of Y93H RAS was also studied in the ALLY 3 study in GT3 cirrhotic patients.[30] Patients with both cirrhosis and Y93H RAS had only a 25% SVR12. Due to these findings, AASLD-IDSA recommends that treatment-naïve cirrhotic patients with HCV GT3 should be treated with sofosbuvir and daclatasvir and RBV for 24 weeks if pretreatment Y93H RASs are present, and RBV may or may not be used if the Y93H RAS is absent.[5] The EASL guidelines recommend 24 weeks of sofosbuvir and daclatasvir with RBV in all cirrhotic patients (regardless of past treatment history); thus, they do not recommend RAS testing in cirrhotic patients receiving this regimen.[6]

This group of treatment-naïve GT3 patients with compensated cirrhosis can also receive sofosbuvir/velpatasvir/voxilaprevir (Vosevi®) as an alternative regimen for 12 weeks when the Y93H RAS is present. The POLARIS-3 study looked at such patients and used 8 weeks of sofosbuvir/velpatasvir/voxilaprevir.[34] The SVR was 96% (106/110). However, due to a concern of a lower SVR rate in patients with the Y93H mutation, the FDA approved this for a 12-week regimen for this indication.

Genotype 3, Treatment-Experienced

The guidelines for treatment-experienced GT3 HCV patients vary based on whether patients had been previous nonresponders to interferon-based therapy or DAA-based regimens. The currently recommended treatments are outlined in Table 10.3.

Genotype 3, Treatment-Experienced to PEG-IFN/RBV, Noncirrhotic

These recommendations are based on the results of the above-mentioned ASTRAL 3 and ALLY 3 and SURVEYOR-2 studies. In the ASTRAL 3 study, patients received 12 weeks of oral sofosbuvir/velpatasvir[22]; 91% of treatment-experienced patients without cirrhosis achieved an SVR12. In the ALLY 3 study, 94% of patients with PEG-IFN/RBV treatment-experienced, noncirrhotic GT3 HCV patients treated with sofosbuvir and daclatasvir for 12 weeks achieved SVR12.[30] As mentioned previously, Y93H RAS had a negative impact on the success of treatment in this group of GT3 HCV patients. Thus, the addition of RBV in treatment-experienced patients with baseline Y93H RAS is recommended.

In the SURVEYOR-2 study of glecaprevir/pibrentasvir, noncirrhotic GT3 3 patients who were treatment-experienced to PEG-IFN and RBV, the SVR rates were 91% (20/22) for 12 weeks of therapy and 96% (21/22) for 16 weeks of therapy.[31] Based on these data, this combination is recommended by AASLD-IDSA as an alternative regimen for 16 weeks in this group of patients.

As noted earlier, based on results of the POLARIS-3 study, the AASLD-IDSA guidelines consider sofosbuvir/velpatasvir/voxilaprevir for 12 weeks as an alternative regimen in this group of patients when the Y93H RAS is present.[34]

Genotype 3, Treatment-Experienced to PEG-IFN/RBV, Compensated Cirrhotic

Sofosbuvir/velpatasvir/voxilaprevir is recommended by AASLD-IDSA for this group of GT-3 patients for 12 weeks based on data from the POLARIS-3 trial.[34]

The C-ISLE study evaluated elbasvir (an NS5A inhibitor) and grazoprevir (a protease inhibitor) and sofosbuvir with and without RBV in this subset of GT-3 patients.[35] The 12-week course without RBV had a 100% SVR (17/17) and is a recommended regimen by AASLD-IDSA.

In the ASTRAL 3 trial, cirrhotic patients treated with sofosbuvir/velpatasvir for 12 weeks achieved SVR12 rates of 89%.[22] Extrapolated data suggested that prolonging the course of this regimen and/or adding RBV would increase the SVR12 rate to greater than 90%. Thus, the AASLD-IDSA and EASL both make these recommendations as outlined in Table 10.3.[5,6]

In the ALLY 3 trial, SVR12 was only achieved in 69% of PEG-IFN/RBV treatment-experienced cirrhotic patients treated with 12 weeks of sofosbuvir and daclatasvir.[30] In the ALLY 3+ study of cirrhotic patients with GT3 HCV, SVR rates were improved to 89% with extension of treatment to 16 weeks and the addition of RBV to the regimen.[31] Given that treatment-experienced compensated cirrhotic GT3 HCV patients represent one of the most difficult to treat groups, EASL recommends prolonging the treatment course of sofosbuvir and daclatasvir and/or adding RBV to increase SVR12 rates as outlined in Table 10.3.[5,6]

In the SURVEYOR-2 study of glecaprevir/pibrentasvir, cirrhotic GT3 patients who were treatment-experienced to PEG-IFN and RBV or sofosbuvir and RBV+/− PEG-IFN, the SVR rates were 96% (45/47) with 16 weeks of therapy.[31]

Genotype 3, Treatment-Experienced to Sofosbuvir and RBV with or Without Cirrhosis

Because of the suboptimal SVR rates with sofosbuvir plus RBV therapy, there are a substantial portion of patients who have failed this regimen. As a result there is a significant unmet need for effective treatment regimens in this population. The recommendations are included in Table 10.3 but are often based on limited data and expert opinion. For example, in the ALLY 3 study, seven patients who had failed sofosbuvir-containing regimens were treated with 12 weeks of sofosbuvir and daclatasvir, with 71% achieving SVR12.[30]

The only recommended regimen through AASLD-IDSA is 12 weeks of sofosbuvir/velpatasvir/voxilaprevir (with the addition of weight-based RBV if the patient had failed a prior NS5A inhibitor and has cirrhosis) based on data from the POLARIS-1 and POLARIS-4 studies.[36]

Given the limited data, the AASLD-IDSA guidance document also suggests considering waiting for newer regimens if there is no immediate or urgent need for treatment.[5] The EASL guidelines have different treatment recommendations based on the degree of fibrosis, as outlined in Table 10.3.[6]

Genotype 3, Decompensated Cirrhosis

The treatment recommendations for decompensated GT3 HCV patients are as outlined in Table 10.3. Again, this is a difficult to treat group with only limited study data available. As noted in the table, these patients will require prolonged therapy and/or the addition of RBV to the regimen.

In the ASTRAL 4 study, the SVR12 rate was 50% for patients treated with sofosbuvir/velpatasvir for 12 weeks, 85% for patients treated with sofosbuvir/velpatasvir and RBV for 12 weeks, and 50% for patients treated with sofosbuvir/velpatasvir for 24 weeks.[27]

In the ALLY 1 study which used sofosbuvir and daclatasvir and weight-based RBV for 12 weeks in patients with advanced cirrhosis, the number of GT3 patients (only 6 patients) was too small to make firm evidence-based recommendations[28]; 83% (5/6) of patients achieved SVR in this group.

In a trial presented at the AASLD Annual Meeting in 2015, the European compassionate use program was described for patients with advanced HCV GT3. In this study, 81% had cirrhosis and 56% were Child's B or C. Using 24 weeks of sofosbuvir and daclatasvir with or without RBV, the SVR rate was 86–88%.[33]

Using a European expanded-access program, Foster et a. showed a 72.8% SVR rate in HCV GT3 patients with decompensated cirrhosis treated with 12 weeks of sofosbuvir and daclatasvir with or without RBV.[32]

Again, note that regimens containing protease inhibitors are not recommended for patients with decompensated cirrhosis.

HCV Genotype 2 and 3 Patients with Renal Failure

As noted earlier, sofosbuvir has not been extensively studied in patients with a CrCl of less than 30 and those on dialysis so dosing cannot be recommended in this population per the manufacturer's recommendations. Studies looking at the safety and efficacy of sofosbuvir-based regimens in these groups are ongoing.

The combination of glecaprevir/pibrentasvir was approved in late 2017. There are no restrictions on the use of this medication for patients with renal failure. Thus, the recommendations for this combination for GT2 and GT3 patients are the same as those in patients with normal renal function.

Conclusion

In the era of direct-acting antivirals for the treatment of hepatitis C, it is clear now that the majority of patients with GT2 and GT3 HCV can be successfully treated with an all-oral regimen. Genotype 2 is more responsive than GT3 to all-oral therapy, perhaps due to accelerated steatosis and fibrosis development seen in patients with GT3. While all-oral therapy can eradicate disease in most patients, some populations may still benefit from the addition of RBV and/or prolongation of the treatment course (especially in treatment-experienced, cirrhotic GT3 patients). There is also a role for resistance testing in many patients with GT3 disease. Given the potential need for RBV in some of the currently approved regimens for genotypes 2 and 3, there remains a need for further drug development in those patients with hematologic comorbidities.

References

1. Messina JP, et al. Global distribution and prevalence of hepatitis C virus genotypes. *Hepatology*. 2015;61:77–87.

2. Alter M, et al. The prevalence of hepatitis C viral infection in the United States, 1988-1994. *N Engl J Med*. 1999;341:556–562.

3. Bochud PY, et al. Genotype 3 is associated with accelerated fibrosis progression in chronic hepatitis C. *J Hepatol*. 2009;51:655–666.

4. Lonardo A, et al. Hepatitis C and steatosis: a reappraisal. *J Viral Hepat*. 2006;13:73–80.

5. American Association for the Study of Liver Diseases, Infections Diseases Society of America. Recommendations for testing, managing and treating hepatitis C. Combined AASLD-IDSA guidelines. www.hcvguidelines.org. Accessed October 20, 2017.

6. European Association for the Study of the Liver. EASL recommendations on treatment of hepatitis C 2016. *J Hepatol*. 2017;66:153–194.

7. Pearlman BL, et al. Sustained virologic response to antiviral therapy for hepatitis C virus infection: a cure and so much more. *Clin Infect Dis*. 2011;52:889–900.

8. Lindsay K. Introduction to therapy of hepatitis C. *Hepatology*. 2002;36(Suppl.1):S114–S120.

9. Backus L, et al. A sustained virologic response reduces risk of all-cause mortality in patients with hepatitis C. *Clin Gastroenterol Hepatol*. 2011;9:509–516.

10. Chen J, et al. Earlier sustained virologic response endpoints for regulatory approval and dose selection of hepatitis C therapies. *Gastroenterology*. 2013;144:1450–455.

11. Fried MW, et al. Peginterferon alfa-2a plus ribavirin for chronic hepatitis C virus infection. *N Engl J Med*. 2002;347:975–982.

12. Manns M, et al. Peginterferon alfa-2b plus ribavirin for initial treatment of chronic hepatitis C: a randomized trial. *Lancet*. 2001;358:959–965.

13. Shoeb D, et al. Extended duration therapy with pegylated-interferon and ribavirin for patients with genotype 3 hepatitis C and advanced fibrosis: final results from the STEPS trial. *J Hepatol*. 2014;60:699–705.

14. Sovaldi (Sofosbuvir) package insert. Gilead Sciences.

15. Epclusa (Sofosbuvir/Velpatasvir) package insert. Gilead Sciences.

16. Daklinza (Daclatasvir) package insert. Bristol-Myers Squibb.

17. Lawitz E, et al. Sofosbuvir for previously untreated hepatitis C infection. *N Engl J Med*. 2013;368:1878–1887.

18. Jacobson IM, et al. Sofosbuvir for hepatitis C genotypes 2 or 3 in patients without treatment options. *N Engl J Med*. 2013;368:1867–1877.

19. Zeuzem S, et al. Sofosbuvir and ribavirin in HCV genotypes 2 and 3. *N Engl J Med*. 2014;370:1993–2001.

20. Lawitz E, et al. Sofosbuvir with pegylated-interferon and ribavirin for 12 weeks in previously treated patients with hepatitis C genotypes 2 or 3 and cirrhosis. *Hepatology*. 2015;61:769–775.

21. Feld JJ, et al. Sofosbuvir and velpatasvir for HCV genotype 1, 2, 4, 5, and 6 infection. *N Engl J Med*. 2015;373:2599–2607.

22. Foster GR, et al. Sofosbuvir and velpatasvir for HCV genotype 2 and 3 infection. *N Engl J Med*. 2015;373:2608–2617.

23. Hassanein T, et al. SURVEYOR-II, Part 4: Glecaprevir/Pibrentasvir demonstrates high SVR rates in patients with HCV genotype 2,4,5 or 6 infection without cirrhosis following an 8-week treatment duration. *Hepatology*;64(suppl S1):XXX.

24. Forns X, et al. Glecaprevir plus pibrentasvir for chronic hepatitis C virus genotype 1,2,4,5 or 6 infection in adults with compensated cirrhosis (EXPEDITION-1): a signle-arm, open-label, multicenter phase 3 trial. *Lancet Infect Dis.* 2017;17:1062–8.

25. Wyles DL, et al. Daclatasvir plus sofosbuvir for HCV in patients coinfected with HIV-1. *N Engl J Med.* 2015;373:714–725.

26. Sulkowski MS, Gardiner DF, Rodriguez-Torres M, et al. Daclatasvir plus sofosbuvir for previously treated and untreated chronic HCV infection. *N Engl J Med.* 2014;370:211–221.

27. Curry MP, et al. Sofosbuvir and velpatasvir for HCV in patients with decompensated cirrhosis. *N Engl J Med.* 2015;373:2618–2628.

28. Poorrad F, et al. Daclatasvir with sofosbuvir and ribavirin for hepatitis C virus infection with advanced cirrhosis or post-liver transplantation recurrence. *Hepatology.* 2016;63:1493–1505.

29. Foster GR, et al. ENDURANCE-3: safety and efficacy of glecaprevir/pibrentasvir compared to sofosbuvir plus daclatasvir in treatment-naïve HCV genotype 3-infected patients without cirrhosis. *J Hepatol.* 2017;66(suppl):GS-007A.

30. Nelson DR, et al. All-oral 12-week treatment with daclatasvir plus sofosbuvir in patients with hepatitis C virus genotype 3 infection: ALLY-3 phase III study. *Hepatology.* 2015;61:1127–1135.

31. Wyles DL, et al. SURVEYOR-II, part 3: efficacy and safety of ABT-493/ABT-530 in patients with hepatitis C virus genotype 3 infection with prior treatment experience and/or cirrhosis. *Hepatology.* 2016;64(suppl S1):62A.

32. Leroy V, et al. Daclatasvir, sofosbuvir, and ribavirin for hepatitis C virus genotype 3 and advanced liver disease: a randomized phase III study (ALLY 3+). *Hepatology.* 2016;63:1430–1441.

33. Welzel TM, et al. Safety and efficacy of daclatasvir plus sofosbuvir with or without ribavirin for the treatment of chronic HCV genotype 3 infection: interim results of a multicenter European compassionate use program. *Hepatology.* 2015;62(suppl S1):225A.

34. Foster GR, et al. A randomized, phase 3 trial of sofosbuvir/velpatasvir/voxilaprevir for 8 weeks and sofosbuvir/velpatasvir for 12 weeks for patients with genotype 3 HCV infection and cirrhosis: the POLARIS-3 study. *Hepatology.* 2016;64(suppl S1):135A.

35. Foster GR, et al. C-ISLE: grazoprevir/elbasvir plus sofosbuvir in treatment-naïve and treatment-experienced HCV GT3 cirrhotic patients treated for 8, 12 or 16 weeks. *Hepatology.* 2016;64(suppl S1):39A.

36. Bourliere M, et al. Sofosbuvir, velpatasvir and voxilaprevir for previously treated HCV infection. *N Engl J Med.* 2017;376:2134–2146.

37. Foster GR, et al. Impact of direct acting antiviral therapy in patients with chronic hepatitis C and decompensated cirrhosis. *J Hepatol.* 2016;64:1224–1231.

Chapter 11

Treatment of Hepatitis C in Special Populations

Andres F. Carrion and Paul Martin

Chronic hepatitis C virus (HCV) infection remains a public health challenge, with an estimated global prevalence of 2.8%, implying that more than 185 million people are infected worldwide, although this is likely an underestimate. The disease is generally slowly progressive and characterized by persistent hepatic inflammation that leads to cirrhosis in approximately 10–20% of individuals over the course of 20–30 years time, with distinct variability in progression based on multiple variables.[1] Once cirrhosis is established, complications such as ascites, variceal hemorrhage, hepatic encephalopathy, hepatocellular carcinoma (HCC), and/or acute on chronic liver failure may develop and diminish quality of life and survival without liver transplantation.

Effective antiviral therapy that results in sustained virological response (SVR) is the only strategy that significantly alters the natural history of liver disease associated with HCV infection by reducing the frequency of hepatic decompensation, liver-related mortality, all-cause mortality, need for liver transplantation, and HCC.[2] Furthermore, SVR is also associated with improved quality of life and increased work productivity.[3] Licensure of new-generation direct-acting antiviral agents (DAAs) revolutionized treatment of HCV infection as these agents have very high virological efficacy, low frequency of severe adverse events (AEs), and overall high barrier to resistance. Nevertheless, important therapeutic challenges remain in specific populations such as individuals with decompensated cirrhosis, advanced-stage chronic kidney disease (CKD), liver transplant recipients, HCV/human immunodeficiency virus (HIV) coinfection, and those who previously failed antiviral therapy for HCV with new-generation DAAs.

Treatment of HCV in Individuals with Decompensated Cirrhosis

Case: A 53-year-old African-American woman with HCV genotype (GT) 1a infection, naïve to antiviral therapy, is being evaluated for treatment. She has decompensated cirrhosis with complications that include history of esophageal variceal hemorrhage treated with endoscopic band ligation and a nonselective β-blocker, ascites that is managed with diuretics and sodium restriction, and hepatic encephalopathy treated with lactulose. Overall, the patient feels well and is able to independently perform activities of daily living. Child-Turcotte-Pugh (CTP) score is 8, class B, and model for end-stage liver disease (MELD) score is 11 (bilirubin 1.4 mg/dL, creatinine 0.8 mg/dL, international normalized ratio [INR] 1.3). Hemoglobin level is 14 g/dL. Her initial visit at a liver transplantation center is scheduled in 1 month. What are the benefits and risks of HCV therapy in patients with decompensated cirrhosis?

Hepatic decompensation results in markedly diminished survival and poor quality of life, thus liver transplantation remains the treatment of choice regardless of the etiology of liver disease. Nevertheless, the large imbalance between potential candidates for liver transplantation and supply of donor organs remains an important limitation. Antiviral therapy with interferon (IFN)-based regimens was particularly challenging in this population due to toxicity and exceedingly poor SVR. In contrast, IFN-free regimens with DAAs have excellent tolerability and high virological efficacy in individuals with decompensated cirrhosis (CTP classes B and C); thus, these agents have renewed interest in treatment of HCV infection in this population.

Prior to initiating antiviral therapy with DAAs in individuals with decompensated cirrhosis it is important to assess and determine potential candidacy for liver transplantation. Conceivable benefits and risks of treating HCV infection pre- versus post-liver transplantation should be discussed in detail. Some important clinical points unique to this population that must be addressed include (1) potential for improvement of biochemical parameters without significant improvement in quality of life following successful antiviral therapy (MELD limbo or purgatory); (2) use of HCV-infected grafts for liver transplantation; and (3) safety, tolerability, and efficacy of DAAs in decompensated cirrhosis compared to post-liver transplantation.

Improvement of hepatic function is commonly observed during and after successful antiviral therapy with DAAs, even in individuals with severe hepatic decompensation (CTP class C), and is mainly reflected by reductions in serum bilirubin and prothrombin time resulting in lower MELD scores.[4,5] Nevertheless, despite reductions in the MELD score following successful antiviral therapy for HCV, individuals may continue to experience poor quality of life and severe complications of cirrhosis. Organ allocation for liver transplantation in most countries is dictated by disease severity models such as the MELD score that incorporate biochemical parameters but not impairment of quality of life; thus, such reductions in biochemical parameters and consequently the MELD score following antiviral therapy for HCV may result in some individuals with poor quality of life due to liver-related complications to fall below the range of contention for organ allocation. This has been termed "MELD limbo or MELD purgatory" and should be a consideration prior to starting antiviral therapy in individuals with decompensated cirrhosis and MELD scores approaching the range in which liver transplantation is a realistic option.[6]

The persistent shortage of donor grafts along with robust data supporting the efficacy and safety of antiviral regimens with DAAs for treatment of recurrent HCV infection in liver transplant recipients has resulted in consideration of use of HCV-infected grafts for individuals with HCV infection listed for liver transplantation. Although no clinical trial to date has evaluated the efficacy of antiviral regimens with DAAs following transplantation of HCV-positive liver grafts, outcomes are expected to be similar compared to treatment of recurrent HCV infection following transplantation of an HCV-negative liver graft. A similar approach has been studied in HCV-infected renal transplant recipients who received a renal graft from an HCV-infected donor and were treated with DAAs post-renal transplantation demonstrating excellent SVR (96%) and tolerability.[7]

DAAs targeting the NS5B (sofosbuvir) and NS5A (ledipasvir, daclatasvir, velpatasvir, pibrentasvir) viral proteins are in general well-tolerated by individuals with decompensated cirrhosis.[4,5] In contrast, NS3/4A protease inhibitors such as simeprevir, grazoprevir, paritaprevir, glecaprevir, and voxilaprevir are contraindicated in this population due to increased drug levels as well as postmarketing reports of worsening hepatic decompensation and liver failure in individuals treated with agents from this class. If no contraindications exist (i.e., anemia), concomitant administration of ribavirin (RBV) is recommended for all individuals with decompensated cirrhosis receiving antiviral therapy with regimens containing DAAs (regardless of the GT) because it enhances SVR. The recommended initial dose for RBV in individuals with severe hepatic decompensation (CTP class C) is 600 mg orally once daily, which can be subsequently increased as tolerated. If RBV is contraindicated, extending the duration of therapy from 12 to 24 weeks is an alternative for all regimens containing DAAs. Table 11.1 summarizes various antiviral regimens currently recommended by guidelines for use in individuals with decompensated cirrhosis.

Antiviral therapy with sofosbuvir (NS5B nucleotide polymerase inhibitor) in combination with an NS5A inhibitor such as ledipasvir, daclatasvir, or velpatasvir along with concomitant RBV for 12 weeks results in SVR in 82–96% of individuals with HCV GT1 infection and decompensated cirrhosis.[4,5,8] In general, SVR rates are higher for GT1b compared to 1a following antiviral therapy with DAAs. CTP class also predicts response to antiviral therapy, with CTP class B demonstrating higher SVR than CTP class C. The combination of sofosbuvir plus either daclatasvir or velpatasvir along with concomitant RBV for treatment of genotypes 2 and 3 results in SVR in 80–100% and 83–85%, respectively.[4,8] Although the number of individuals enrolled in clinical trials with GT4 and decompensated cirrhosis has been modest, reported SVR following treatment with sofosbuvir plus ledipasvir, daclatasvir, or velpatasvir with concomitant RBV is 67–100%.[4,5,8]

Table 11.1 Antiviral regimens with direct-acting antiviral agents (DAAs) recommended for individuals with hepatic decompensation

DAAs	HCV Genotypes	Duration	
		DAAs plus RBV	DAAs without RBV
Sofosbuvir/ledipasvir	1, 4	12 weeks	24 weeks
Sofosbuvir/daclatasvir	1, 2, 3	12 weeks	24 weeks
Sofosbuvir/velpatasvir	1, 2, 3, 4, 5, 6	12 weeks	24 weeks

Antiviral regimens containing sofosbuvir, an NS5A inhibitor (ledipasvir, daclatasvir, or velpatasvir), and RBV are associated with universal occurrence of AEs in individuals with decompensated cirrhosis, but they are most typically mild, such as fatigue, gastrointestinal intolerance, anemia, and headache. Nevertheless, more severe AEs occur in 11–42% of individuals with decompensated cirrhosis resulting in discontinuation of DAAs in up to 8%. Mortality during or shortly after completion of antiviral therapy has been reported in up to 3% of treated individuals.[4,5,8]

Improvement of hepatic function reflected by reduction in CTP or MELD scores has been reported in up to 60% of individuals who achieve SVR and is more noticeable in those with higher baseline scores (81% of patients with MELD score ≥15 vs. 51% of patients with MELD score <15).[4,5,8] Whether these improvements persist long term remain to be documented; nevertheless, a recent population-based study showed a 32% decline in liver transplantation listings for HCV-related liver disease during 2014–2015 compared to previous years.[9]

In summary, availability of IFN-free regimens with DAAs permits treatment of HCV in individuals with decompensated cirrhosis with overall high virological efficacy across different genotypes. Importantly, SVR rates are in general lower in individuals with decompensated cirrhosis (CTP classes B and C) compared to those seen in individuals with compensated cirrhosis (CTP class A) and liver transplant recipients (with or without cirrhosis but no hepatic decompensation). Furthermore, the frequency of AEs (including severe AEs) is markedly higher in this population; thus, selection of candidates with hepatic decompensation for antiviral therapy must be judicious. The patient presented in the vignette has a low MELD score and overall no significant impairment of daily activities or quality of life. Improvement of hepatic function following antiviral therapy is anticipated and may contribute to further improvement of overall health without compromising candidacy for liver transplantation based on an already low MELD score. Antiviral therapy with sofosbuvir plus an NS5A inhibitor (ledipasvir, daclatasvir, or velpatasvir) with concomitant RBV for 12 weeks should be used and high SVR is expected.

Treatment of HCV in Individuals with Advanced CKD

Case: A 48-year-old Caucasian man is evaluated for treatment of HCV GT1a naïve to antiviral therapy. He has advanced CKD due to diabetic nephropathy with a serum creatinine level of 7.3 mg/dL and an estimated glomerular filtration rate (eGFR) of 8 mL/min/1.73 m^2 requiring hemodialysis thrice weekly. He has no clinical features to suggest cirrhosis, platelet count is 230,000/μL, and other biochemical parameters reflect preserved synthetic function. Liver stiffness measurement estimated by transient elastography is 5 kPa (F0–F1). He had been previously told that he was not a "good treatment candidate" for sofosbuvir-based antiviral regimens due to renal disease. Is this individual a candidate for treatment with any other DAAs?

The prevalence of HCV infection in individuals with CKD receiving renal replacement therapy varies significantly in different countries: 2.7–3.9% in the United Kingdom and Germany, 7.5–14% in the United States, and as high as 80% in countries such as Morocco, Moldavia, and Egypt.[10] Nosocomial transmission within hemodialysis units remains the most important risk factor for infection in this population, with the risk being proportional to the prevalence of HCV within individual hemodialysis units and time on hemodialysis.[11] HCV infection in individuals with CKD is associated with increased morbidity and mortality compared to noninfected controls with similar impairment of renal function. This difference may reflect faster progression to cirrhosis with a higher incidence of complications of cirrhosis, including HCC, as well as increased risk of extrahepatic comorbidities such as cardiovascular events.[12,13] HCV infection is also associated with adverse outcomes in renal transplant recipients, including inferior patient and graft survival rates as well as increased risk for graft nephropathy, new-onset diabetes after transplantation, and sepsis.[14]

Individuals with CKD were until recently a very challenging population for treatment of HCV due to the toxicity and low efficacy of IFN- and RBV-based regimens. RBV is poorly tolerated in this population (even low doses) because anemia is prevalent at baseline (up to 70% in individuals with CKD stage 5).[15] Despite availability of several IFN-free regimens containing DAAs that have proved to be safe and effective in individuals with mild to moderate CKD (eGFR ≥30 mL/min/1.73 m^2), specific challenges remain in clinical practice for those with more advanced stages of renal disease because some DAAs undergo extensive renal clearance (Table 11.2).

Sofosbuvir is predominantly renally excreted (80%), and accumulation of its metabolite GS-331007 occurs in severe CKD; thus, this agent is only licensed for use in individuals with eGFR of 30 mL/min/1.73 m^2 or greater. Following a single dose of 400 mg, the area under the curve (AUC) of sofosbuvir and GS-331007 is 171% and 451% higher, respectively, in individuals with an eGFR of less than 30 mL/min/1.73m^2 compared to those with normal renal function. Dialysis removes only a small proportion of sofosbuvir (18%) and its

Table 11.2 Renal excretion of licensed direct-acting antiviral agents (DAAs)

DAAs	Renal Excretion
Sofosbuvir	80%
Simeprevir	<1%
Daclatasvir	6.6%
Ledipasvir	<1%
Velpatasvir	<1%
Pibrentasvir	0%
PrOD	1.9–11.3%
Elbasvir/grazoprevir	<1%
Voxilaprevir	0%
Glecaprevir	<1%

PrOD, paritaprevir, ritonavir, ombitasvir, and dasabuvir.

metabolite. Relative to individuals with normal renal function, following a single dose 1 hour before hemodialysis, the AUC of sofosbuvir and GS-331007 is 28% and 1280% higher, respectively, and 60% and 2070% higher, respectively, when a single dose is administered 1 hour after hemodialysis. Several groups have studied the safety and efficacy of sofosbuvir at various dosages (400 mg orally daily, 200 mg orally daily, or 400 mg orally every other day) in combination with simeprevir for treatment of GT1 infection in individuals with an eGFR of less than 30 mL/min/1.73m^2. Although data are limited to small series, reported SVR rates range between 80% and 100% following 12 weeks of sofosbuvir and simeprevir with or without concomitant low-dose RBV.[16–18] Initial experience with sofosbuvir in advanced-stage CKD is encouraging; nevertheless, further data are required before this agent's use outside clinical trials can be endorsed if the eGFR is less than 30 mL/min/1.73m^2.

NS3/4A protease inhibitors such as simeprevir, paritaprevir, grazoprevir, glecaprevir, and voxilaprevir are primarily excreted by the liver with minimal renal clearance. As mentioned earlier, simeprevir has been studied in combination with various dosages of sofosbuvir in individuals with advanced CKD, but data are limited to small series.[16,17] Paritaprevir is part of the multidrug regimen that also contains low-dose ritonavir and ombitasvir with or without dasabuvir (PrOD). This regimen is one of three currently licensed for treatment of HCV genotypes 1 (with dasabuvir) and 4 (without dasabuvir) in individuals with mild, moderate, and severe CKD, including those on hemodialysis. Although increased AUC of dasabuvir (50%), paritaprevir (45%), and ritonavir (114%) occurs in individuals with severe renal impairment (eGFR <30 mL/min/1.73m^2), no significant increase in AEs has been described in this population compared to individuals with normal renal function. Data from one small study showed 90% SVR in individuals with GT1 infection and eGFR of less than 30 mL/min/1.73m^2, including 70% on hemodialysis treated with 12 weeks of PrOD.[19] Concomitant low-dose RBV (200 mg orally daily) was used for individuals with GT1a infection only. AEs were common (50%) and mainly related to RBV; severe anemia requiring interruption and/or discontinuation of this agent occurred in 69% of individuals. Severe AEs occurred in 20%, but the single death following completion of therapy was thought to be unrelated to DAAs or RBV. Grazoprevir is coformulated as single tablet with the NS5A inhibitor elbasvir. This regimen was studied in a large, randomized, placebo-controlled trial that enrolled individuals with HCV GT1 infection and an eGFR of less than 30 mL/min/1.73m^2, including 76% on hemodialysis. Elbasvir/grazoprevir was administered for 12 weeks without RBV, and SVR was 99%. Importantly, this trial had a placebo arm (deferred treatment group) permitting accurate safety evaluation with no significant difference in frequency of AEs between the immediate and deferred treatment groups.[20] Baseline testing for NS5A resistance-associated variants (RAVs) is recommended prior to elbasvir/grazoprevir therapy for GT1a. In the presence of baseline RAVs, lengthening therapy from 12 to 16 weeks and using concomitant RBV is advisable. Nevertheless, to date, SVR rates have been similar in individuals with advanced stages of CKD with and without these polymorphisms treated with standard 12 weeks of elbasvir/grazoprevir without RBV. Glecaprevir/pibrentasvir was recently licensed as a pan-genotypic antiviral regimen. Both agents are primarily excreted by the liver with minimal renal clearance; thus, this regimen can be used in individuals with advanced CKD, including those undergoing hemodialysis.[21]

NS5A inhibitors such as ledipasvir, daclatasvir, ombitasvir, velpatasvir, and pibrentasvir are primarily metabolized by the liver with only minimal renal excretion (Table 11.2) and no clinically significant difference in pharmacokinetics has been noted in individuals with an eGFR of less than 30 mL/min/1.73m^2 compared to those with an eGFR of 30 mL/min/1.73m^2 or higher. Ledipasvir, daclatasvir, and velpatasvir are, however, licensed only in combination with sofosbuvir, which is indicated for individuals with an eGFR of 30 mL/min/1.73m^2 or higher.

Antiviral regimens for treatment of HCV genotypes 2, 3, 5, and 6 containing sofosbuvir should not be used in individuals with an eGFR of less than 30 mL/min/1.73m^2. The only regimen currently licensed to treat these genotypes in advanced CKD including hemodialysis is glecaprevir/pibrentasvir.

Individuals with decompensated cirrhosis and advanced CKD remain a challenging population for HCV therapy even with currently available DAAs. Sofosbuvir is not recommended if the eGFR is less than 30 mL/min/1.73m^2, and protease inhibitors are contraindicated due to severe hepatic dysfunction. These patients should be referred to a transplant center for consideration of combined liver-kidney transplantation.

In summary, HCV infection in individuals with CKD results in diminished survival due to hepatic and extrahepatic complications and also impairs recipient and graft survival following renal transplantation. The benefits of successful antiviral therapy in this population are substantial and include reduction of complications related to liver disease and cardiovascular morbidity, as well as the likelihood of graft injury following renal transplantation. Individuals with an eGFR of 30 mL/min/1.73m^2 or higher may be treated with any of the currently licensed regimens, but those with an eGFR of less than 30 mL/min/1.73m^2 should not receive sofosbuvir-based regimens. Elbasvir/grazoprevir, PrOD (with low-dose RBV for GT1a), and glecaprevir/pibrentasvir are safe and effective regimens for treatment of HCV in individuals without cirrhosis and those with compensated cirrhosis (CTP class A) with an eGFR of less than 30 mL/min/1.73m^2, including those on hemodialysis. The patient in the clinical vignette represented up until recently a major therapeutic dilemma; nevertheless, elbasvir/grazoprevir or glecaprevir/pibrentasvir are highly effective and safe RBV-free regimen for treatment of GT1a in advanced CKD.[20,21]

Recurrent HCV Infection in Liver Transplant Recipients

Case: A 61-year-old Hispanic man underwent liver transplantation 2 years ago for decompensated cirrhosis. He has had HCV GT3 infection for more than 20 years and is treatment naïve. Persistent elevation of the aminotransferases following liver transplantation has led to several liver biopsies all showing chronic inflammation without convincing evidence of rejection. The most recent biopsy showed grade 3 inflammatory activity and METAVIR stage 2 fibrosis. Renal function is normal. Hemoglobin level is 14.2 g/dL. Medications include tacrolimus, mycophenolate mofetil, and amlodipine. What is the role of antiviral therapy in this patient?

Recurrent HCV infection occurs almost invariably in liver transplant recipients (with detectable viremia at the time of transplantation) with an accelerated course resulting in reduction in patient and graft survival.[22] Recurrent HCV is responsible for 25–30% of all hepatic graft losses, and cirrhosis and overt hepatic decompensation occurs in approximately one-third of liver transplant recipients within 5 years posttransplant, rising to 50% at 10 years.[23] In contrast, individuals who achieve SVR prior to liver transplantation do not develop recurrent HCV infection and have outcomes comparable to other indications for liver transplantation.[24]

Antiviral therapy for HCV in liver transplant recipients previously presented unique challenges. IFN-based regimens were in general contraindicated in solid-organ transplant recipients due to high risk for rejection. Liver transplant recipients were, however, considered an exception, and IFN was used in selected cases as a measure to preserve hepatic function and arrest progressive fibrosis leading to graft dysfunction. Fibrosing cholestatic hepatitis is an uncommon but severe and rapidly progressive form of liver injury occasionally seen in liver transplant recipients with recurrent HCV infection.[25,26]

New-generation DAAs are highly effective, safe, and well-tolerated following liver transplantation. Multiple IFN-free regimens have been studied in liver transplant recipients and include sofosbuvir/simeprevir (GT1), sofosbuvir/ledipasvir (GT1, 4, 5, 6), sofosbuvir/daclatasvir (GT1, 2, 3, 4), PrOD (GT1), and glecaprevir/pibrentasvir (GT1, 2, 3, 4, 5, 6). Other regimens such as sofosbuvir/velpatasvir, sofosbuvir/velpatasvir/voxilaprevir, and elbasvir/grazoprevir have not been studied in this population. In general, concomitant use of RBV is indicated in liver transplant recipients receiving antiviral regimens with DAAs for 12 weeks (except for glecaprevir/pibrentasvir) because it enhances SVR. Lengthening therapy with DAAs from 12 to 24 weeks should be considered in liver transplant recipients who are RBV ineligible.

Similar to the nontransplant setting, increasing severity of hepatic decompensation in liver transplant recipients with recurrent HCV diminishes SVR. For instance, 12 weeks of sofosbuvir/ledipasvir and RBV for treatment of GT1 infection resulted in SVR in 96% of liver transplant recipients with no cirrhosis or CTP class A, 85% in CTP class B, and 60% in CTP class C.[5]

Antiviral regimens with DAAs with or without concomitant RBV are safe and well-tolerated by liver transplant recipients. The frequency of AEs, including severe AEs and discontinuation of DAAs due to AEs, are similar pre- versus post-liver transplantation when individuals with similar CTP classes are compared. Drug–drug interactions are an important concern in liver transplant recipients and must be anticipated (Table 11.3). Immunosuppressant blood levels and liver chemistries should be closely monitored in this population during and after completion of antiviral therapy with DAAs.

Table 11.3 Potential clinically significant drug–drug interactions between direct-acting antiviral agents (DAAs) and immunosuppressants commonly used in liver transplantation

	Sofosbuvir	Simeprevir	Ledipasvir	Daclatasvir	PrOD	Elbasvir/grazoprevir	Glecaprevir/pibrentasvir
Cyclosporine	No	Yes	Potential	No	Potential	Yes	Yes
Tacrolimus	No	Potential	Potential	No	Potential	Potential	No
Mycophenolate	No	No	No	No	Potential	No	No
Sirolimus	No	Potential	Potential	No	Potential	Potential	Yes
Everolimus	No	Potential	Potential	Potential	Yes	Potential	Yes

PrOD, paritaprevir, ritonavir, ombitasvir, and dasabuvir.

In summary, recurrent HCV infection following liver transplantation results in adverse outcomes including diminished patient and graft survival. Successful antiviral therapy in this population improves survival and reduces hepatic and extrahepatic complications; thus, treatment with DAAs should be attempted in the absence of major contraindications. New-generation DAAs allow for IFN-free regimens that are safe and highly effective in liver transplant recipients. Drug–drug interactions, particularly with immunosuppressant agents, must be anticipated and monitored closely during the course of antiviral therapy. The patient described in the clinical vignette should be promptly treated with an antiviral regimen containing sofosbuvir/daclatasvir (12 weeks with RBV or 24 weeks without RBV) or glecaprevir/pibrentasvir (12 weeks) to arrest inflammatory activity and progressive fibrosis due to HCV. No changes in immunosuppression should be anticipated based on the lack of predicted drug–drug interactions between either antiviral regimen with tacrolimus and mycophenolate mofetil, but close follow-up of tacrolimus blood levels is advisable during and after antiviral therapy.

HCV and HIV Coinfection

Case: A 38-year-old Asian woman with HIV infection diagnosed 8 years ago is evaluated for treatment of HCV GT1a infection naïve to antiviral therapy. HIV is well controlled (CD4$^+$ cell count is 800/μL and undetectable HIV-RNA) with antiretroviral therapy (ART) that includes elvitegravir, cobicistat, emtricitabine, and tenofovir alafenamide. She has no other medical comorbidities. Hepatitis B serologies indicate previous immunization, serum aminotransferases are normal, and there is no evidence of decompensated liver disease. HCV RNA is 12,500,000 IU/mL, and hepatic fibrosis as estimated by transient elastography is F3. What is the role of anti-HCV therapy in individuals with HCV/HIV coinfection?

Approximately 8% of individuals with HCV infection in the United States are coinfected with HIV. In contrast, the proportion of individuals with HIV who have serologic evidence of HCV coinfection is 30%.[27] Coinfection with hepatitis B virus (HBV) occurs in 4.5–8% of HIV-infected individuals in the United States, and triple infection with HCV, HBV, and HIV is less common (1.6%).[28,29] Coinfection reflects shared routes of transmission; therefore, individuals infected with any of these three viruses should be screened for the other two.

Progression from acute to chronic HCV infection occurs more frequently in individuals with HCV/HIV coinfection than in those with HCV monoinfection: 92–95% versus 70–85%, respectively.[30] Coinfection with HCV/HIV is also associated with higher HCV RNA levels, a twofold greater risk of progression to cirrhosis, and a sixfold greater risk of liver failure compared to HCV monoinfection.[31] Liver disease is the most frequent non–HIV-related cause of death in this population, with HCV infection being the most common etiology (66.1%), followed by HBV (16.9%) and HCV/HBV coinfection (7.1%).[32] The risk of HCC is fivefold higher among individuals with coinfection and may occur at a younger age, with a shorter duration of HCV infection, and has a more aggressive course than in individuals with HCV monoinfection.[33,34] Importantly, SVR significantly reduces overall mortality, liver-related mortality, and hepatic decompensation in individuals with HCV/HIV coinfection.[35]

Current HIV treatment guidelines recommend to initiate ART in individuals with HCV coinfection, regardless of the CD4[+] cell count (http://aidsinfo.nih.gov). Correction of severe immunodeficiency (absolute CD4[+] cell count <200/μL) with ART should be attempted prior to starting antiviral therapy for HCV. It may also be appropriate to delay HCV therapy for 1 or 2 months after initiation of ART so the initial AEs of these two regimens are not simultaneous. ART has no direct antiviral effect on HCV, thus HCV RNA levels usually remain unchanged.[34]

In the past, IFN-based regimens resulted in lower SVR and a higher frequency of AEs in individuals with HCV/HIV coinfection compared to those with HCV monoinfection. Nevertheless, antiviral regimens with DAAs have demonstrated high efficacy in this population, with SVR rates that are comparable to those seen in HCV monoinfection. Efficacy of regimens containing DAAs for treatment of various HCV genotypes in individuals with HIV coinfection is summarized in Table 11.4. Selection of a particular regimen for

Table 11.4 Efficacy of direct-acting antiviral agents (DAAs) for treatment of various HCV genotypes in individuals with HIV coinfection

HCV Genotype	DAAs	Duration	SVR
1	Sofosbuvir/ledipasvir	12 weeks	96%
	Sofosbuvir/velpatasvir	12 weeks	95%
	Sofosbuvir/daclatasvir	12 weeks	97%
	PrOD	12 weeks	94%
	Grazoprevir/elbasvir	12 or 16 weeks[a]	94%
	Sofosbuvir/simeprevir	12 weeks	80–90%
	Glecaprevir/pibrentasvir	8, 12, or 16 weeks	100%
2	Sofosbuvir/velpatasvir	12 weeks	100%
	Sofosbuvir/RBV	12 or 16 weeks	89%
	Glecaprevir/pibrentasvir	8 or 12 weeks	100%
3	Sofosbuvir/velpatasvir	12 weeks	92%
	Sofosbuvir/daclatasvir	12 weeks	100%
	Glecaprevir/pibrentasvir	8, 12, or 16 weeks	96%
4	Sofosbuvir/ledipasvir	12 weeks	100%
	Grazoprevir/elbasvir	12 weeks	96%
	Glecaprevir/pibrentasvir	8 or 12 weeks	100%

[a]Twelve weeks of grazoprevir/elbasvir for patients with HCV genotype 1b or 1a infection without NS5A resistance-associated variants (RAVs), 16 weeks with concomitant RBV for patients with positive RAVs. Eight weeks of glecaprevir/pibrentasvir for treatment-naïve patients without cirrhosis and genotypes 1 thru 6 and those without cirrhosis previously treated with regimens containing IFN, RBV, and/or sofosbuvir and genotypes 1, 2, 4, 5, or 6; twelve weeks for treatment naïve patients with compensated cirrhosis and genotypes 1 thru 6, genotype 1 and previous treatment experience with a protease inhibitor.

HCV depends on genotype, hepatic decompensation, previous use of DAAs, and renal function.

Sofosbuvir has very limited drug–drug interactions with agents used as part of ART regimens. Diminished levels of sofosbuvir and its dominant metabolite GS-331007 are expected when used along with ritonavir-boosted tipranavir due to induction of the P-glycoprotein transporter; thus, this combination is not recommended as it may compromise antiviral activity against HCV. Based on data from clinical trials, there are no other significant drug–drug interactions between sofosbuvir and other antiretroviral agents such as tenofovir disoproxil fumarate, emtricitabine, efavirenz, atazanavir, darunavir, raltegravir, and rilpivirine. Similarly, although not based on data from clinical trials but rather from pharmacokinetic properties of individual agents, no drug–drug interactions are expected between sofosbuvir and abacavir, dolutegravir, elvitegravir, and tenofovir alafenamide.[36] Coadministration of ledipasvir or velpatasvir and tenofovir disoproxil fumarate results in elevated levels of the later agent, increasing the risk of renal toxicity. This interaction does not occur with concurrent use of ledipasvir and tenofovir alafenamide. There are no data for drug–drug interactions between ledipasvir and antiretroviral agents including ritonavir-boosted protease inhibitors. Daclatasvir is the only agent that requires dose adjustment based on CYP3A4 induction or inhibition by other drugs. The usual dose is 60 mg orally once daily, but reduction to 30 mg orally once daily is indicated when used concomitantly with ritonavir- or cobicistat-boosted atazanavir. In contrast, a dose increase of daclatasvir to 90 mg orally once daily is required when used concomitantly with efavirenz. Ritonavir (part of the PrOD regimen) results in considerable drug–drug interactions with antiretroviral agents due to strong inhibition of CYP450; thus, PrOD should not be used concurrently with darunavir, efavirenz, rilpivirine, and lopinavir-ritonavir. Major interactions between elbasvir/grazoprevir and antiretroviral agents that preclude concomitant use include efavirenz, etravirine, darunavir, atazanavir, and cobicistat-containing regimens. Glecaprevir/pibrentasvir is contraindicated in patients taking atazanavir due to increased risk of aminotransferase elevations. Increased levels of glacaprevir and pibreantasvir occur when used concurrently with darunavir, lopinavir, or ritonavir; thus, coadministration is not recommended. Coadminstration with efavirenz is also not recommended as it results in diminished levels of gleprevir and pibreantasvir.

Ribavirin-induced hemolytic anemia occurs with higher frequency and is more severe in individuals with HCV/HIV coinfection. This complication is of particular concern when zidovudine is used as part of ART regimens as this agent inhibits the hematopoietic response to RBV-induced hemolysis. Concurrent use of RBV and didanosine is contraindicated as it may result in severe mitochondrial toxicity leading to lactic acidosis, pancreatitis, myopathy, neuropathy, hepatic failure, and death.[37]

In summary, individuals with HCV/HIV coinfection have increased morbidity and mortality from liver disease compared to those with monoinfection with either virus, thus there are compelling reasons to treat HCV in this population. SVR is associated with better outcomes in HCV/HIV coinfection, including diminished liver-related mortality and hepatic decompensation.

Currently licensed IFN-free antiviral regimens containing DAAs have comparable efficacy in individuals with HCV/HIV coinfection and HCV monoinfection. Nevertheless, important drug–drug interactions between DAAs and antiretroviral agents exist and should be carefully accounted when selecting a specific regimen to be used. Furthermore, the decision to treat HCV in these individuals should be a joint one between hepatologist and the infectious disease specialist involved in treatment of HIV. Specific modifications of the ART may be required prior to starting DAAs, and close monitoring for AEs is mandatory during therapy. The patient described in the clinical vignette could receive treatment for HCV with sofosbuvir/ledipasvir, sofosbuvir/velpatasvir, or glecaprevir/pibrentasvir without predicted drug–drug interactions with ART (elvitegravir, cobicistat, emtricitabine, and tenofovir alafenamide). If daclatasvir were to be used in combination with sofosbuvir, dose reduction to 30 mg orally daily is required due to CYP3A4 inhibition by cobicistat. Although PrOD is highly effective for treatment of HCV GT1 in individuals with HIV coinfection, this regimen has significant drug–drug interactions with various antiretroviral agents and, in this particular case, with cobicistat (contraindicated) and elvitegravir (not recommended), thus should not be used. Similarly, elbasvir/grazoprevir is also an effective alternative for treatment of GT1 infection in individuals with HIV but should not be used concomitantly with cobicistat-containing ART regimens.

Retreatment of HCV in Individuals Who Failed Previous Antiviral Regimens

Case: A 48-year-old Hispanic man with HCV GT1a infection relapsed following 12 weeks of antiviral therapy with sofosbuvir/ledipasvir. He had undetectable HCV RNA during and at the end of treatment; nevertheless, HCV RNA was 6,200,000 IU/mL 12 weeks following completion of antiviral therapy. He was compliant with the antiviral regimen, did not miss any dose, and did not take other medications or over-the-counter supplements that could have interacted with DAAs. He had never received antiviral therapy for HCV previously and has compensated cirrhosis (CTP class A) with a MELD score of 7. Renal function is normal and hemoglobin is 14 g/dL. Retreatment with a different antiviral regimen is being contemplated, and testing for NS5A RAVs demonstrated Y93H polymorphism. What antiviral regimen will be advisable for this patient?

Resistance to antiviral agents was initially reported following treatment with the first-generation protease inhibitors boceprevir and telaprevir and has become an important issue in clinical practice for newer generation DAAs. There are two important virological determinants for antiviral resistance: (1) the genetic barrier to resistance, which is the number of nucleotide changes required for the virus to become resistant to specific DAAs; and (2) viral fitness, which is the relative capacity of a viral variant to replicate in a given environment.[38] RAVs are single nucleotide polymorphisms that can be present at baseline (prior to starting antiviral therapy) or emerge during a course of antiviral therapy. These polymorphisms affect the main viral targets for DAAs including NS3/4A, NS5B, and NS5A. In general, NS5A inhibitors (ledipasvir, daclatasvir, ombitasvir, elbasvir, velpatasvir, and pibrentasvir) and NS5B non-nucleoside polymerase inhibitors (dasabuvir) have low barrier to resistance (GT1a lower barrier than GT1b), new generation NS3/4A protease inhibitors (paritaprevir, grazoprevir, glecaprevir, and voxilaprevir) have medium to high barrier to resistance, and the NS5B nucleotide polymerase inhibitor sofosbuvir has high barrier to resistance (Table 11.5).

RAVs existent at baseline are relatively replication unfit, thus typically difficult to detect with conventional assays. During a course of antiviral therapy with DAAs, virions that possess RAVs are suppressed but not eliminated and remain "dormant" in the host as the wild-type virions are eradicated. Once antiviral therapy is discontinued upon completion of therapy, the virions with RAVs that were "selected" during therapy may replicate without competition from wild-type virions that were eradicated, thus resulting in posttreatment virological relapse.

RAVs can be detected with commercially available blood-based assays; nevertheless, universal testing prior to starting antiviral therapy is currently not indicated. A selective approach that takes into account previous treatment failure and choice of DAAs to be used is recommended for deciding when to test for RAVs. For instance, testing is suggested in all individuals who failed a previous antiviral regimen with DAAs in the same class as one that is to be administered in the new regimen. Baseline testing for the Q80K polymorphism (an NS3 RAV) should be obtained prior to starting a regimen containing simeprevir for HCV GT1, and baseline testing for NS5A RAVs is indicated in all individuals with GT1a infection (treatment-naïve or treatment-experienced) who will receive elbasvir/grazoprevir. Current guidelines also suggest considering testing for NS5A RAVs prior to starting therapy with

Table 11.5 Virological resistance to new-generation direct-acting antiviral agents (DAAs)

	NS3/4A Protease Inhibitors	NS5B Nucleotide Polymerase Inhibitors	NS5B Nonnucleoside Polymerase Inhibitors	NS5A Inhibitors
DAAs	Simeprevir Paritaprevir Grazoprevir Glecaprevir Voxilaprevir	Sofosbuvir	Dasabuvir	Ledipasvir Ombitasvir Daclatasvir Elbasvir Velpatasvir Pibrentasvir
Barrier to resistance	Medium	High	Very low	Low
Genotype 1 subtype	1a lower barrier than 1b	No difference	1a lower barrier than 1b	1a lower barrier than 1b

daclatasvir in individuals with GT1a infection. Because the presence of NS5A RAVs does not alter treatment duration with the recently licensed regimens glecaprevir/pibrentasvir and sofosbuvir/velpatasvir/voxilaprevir, testing is not indicated.

Clinical trials have reported baseline prevalence of RAVs: 32–43.6% of individuals with HCV GT1 infection (up to three times more common in GT1a than GT1b) have NS3 RAVs, and 10–14.8% have NS5A RAVs.[20,39-41] In contrast to NS3 RAVs, long-term persistence of NS5A RAVs appears to be more likely as viral fitness is less impaired (Table 11.6).[42] NS5A RAVs are particularly important in individuals with GT1a infection as they are associated with reductions in SVR following treatment with regimens containing some NS5A inhibitors, but their presence at baseline does not alter SVR in individuals with GT1b infection.[42] Selection of RAVs following therapy with the nucleotide polymerase inhibitor sofosbuvir is uncommon and, with the exception of a few reported cases, these have not presented challenges in clinical practice.

In general, when considering retreatment of HCV in individuals who previously failed DAAs, presence of RAVs may guide selection of the new antiviral regimen. Duration of therapy with most DAAs should be extended to 24 weeks and concomitant administration of weight-based RBV (if not contraindicated) is recommended. Exceptions to these rules include elbasvir/grazoprevir, which is recommended for 16 weeks with concomitant RBV for individuals with GT1a and NS5A RAVs; glecaprevir/pibrentasvir, which is recommended for 16 weeks for individuals with GT1 previously treated with an NS5A inhibitor; and, sofosbuvir/velpatasvir/voxilaprevir, which is recommended for 12 weeks without RBV for genotypes 1, 2, 3, 4, 5, and 6.[43,44] Using three DAAs with different mechanisms of action (i.e., NS5B nucleotide or nonnucleoside polymerase inhibitor, NS5A inhibitor, and NS3/4A protease inhibitor) is an attractive option for retreatment of individuals who failed previous regimens with DAAs, and is available with sofosbuvir/velpatasvir/voxilaprevir, which is licensed for retreatment of patients with HCV GT1–6 who failed a previous regimen containing an NS5A inhibitor. This regimen was recently studied in patients with HCV GT1 who failed a previous regimen containing an NS5A inhibitor and in patients with GT1–4 who failed a previous DAA regimen but not an NS5A inhibitor. Following 12 weeks of treatment with sofosbuvir/velpatasvir/voxilaprevir, SVR was achieved in 96% and 98% of patients who previously failed treatment with an antiviral regimen containing an NS5A inhibitor or a DAA regimen not containing an NS5A inhibitor, respectively.[44] Because this regimen contains sofosbuvir and the protease inhibitor voxilaprevir, it is

Table 11.6 Persistence of different resistance-associated variants (RAVs) following treatment with direct-acting antiviral agents (DAAs)

RAVs	24 Weeks Post-Therapy	48 Weeks Post-Therapy
NS3	46%	9%
NS5A	97%	96%

contraindicated in patients with an eGFR of less than 30 mL/min/1.73m^2 and in those with decompensated cirrhosis, respectively.

Glecaprevir/pibrentasvir with or without RBV was also recently studied in a small number of patients with HCV GT1 who failed previous treatment with an antiviral regimen containing an NS5A inhibitor. SVR was achieved in 92% of patients following 12 weeks of antiviral therapy. Among the two virological failures, one patient was treated without RBV, had baseline RAVs for NS3 and NS5A, developed treatment-emergent RAVs, and experienced virological breakthrough during treatment despite having antiviral levels within therapeutic range. The other patient relapsed posttreatment, had baseline NS5A RAVs, and developed treatment-emergent NS3 and NS5A RAVs, despite therapeutic antiviral levels during therapy and concomitant use of RBV.[45]

In summary, although the proportion of individuals who fail antiviral regimens with new-generation DAAs is small, they represent a growing cohort that presents important retreatment challenges. RAVs are single nucleotide polymorphisms of the main virological targets of DAAs that can be present at baseline or emerge during treatment with antiviral agents. The patient presented in the clinical vignette should be treated with 12 weeks of sofosbuvir/velpatasvir/voxilaprevir or 16 weeks of glecaprevir/pibrentasvir, which are the two antiviral regimens currently licensed for retreatment of patients who failed previous antiviral regimen containing an NS5A inhibitor and high SVR is to be expected.

Conclusion

New-generation DAAs are highly effective and well-tolerated in various clinical scenarios and have dramatically changed the landscape of HCV therapeutics. IFN-based regimens were associated with significant toxicity and poor SVR, particularly in selected populations, thus giving birth to the term "special populations for HCV treatment." Nevertheless, specific circumstances in which antiviral therapy with new-generation DAAs remain challenging are few. Some populations that require special attention in this new era of HCV therapeutics include individuals with decompensated cirrhosis because some specific DAAs are associated with increased severe AEs, advanced stage CKD because sofosbuvir is predominantly renally cleared, and liver transplant recipients and HCV/HIV coinfection primarily because of drug–drug interactions. Recently licensed antiviral regimens such as sofosbuvir/velpatasvir/voxilaprevir and glecaprevir/pibrentasvir demonstrate high virological efficacy for retreatment of HCV in individuals who previously failed antiviral regimens containing DAAs.

References

1. Westbrook RH, Dusheiko G. Natural history of hepatitis C. *J Hepatol*. 2014;61:S58–S68.
2. van der Meer AJ, Veldt BJ, Feld JJ, et al. Association between sustained virological response and all-cause mortality among patients with chronic hepatitis C and advanced hepatic fibrosis. *JAMA*. 2012;308:2584–2593.

3. Smith-Palmer J, Cerri K, Valentine W. Achieving sustained virologic response in hepatitis C: a systematic review of the clinical, economic and quality of life benefits. *BMC Infect Dis*. 2015;15:19.

4. Curry MP, O'Leary JG, Bzowej N, et al. Sofosbuvir and velpatasvir for HCV in patients with decompensated cirrhosis. *N Engl J Med*. 2015;373:2618–2628.

5. Charlton M, Everson GT, Flamm SL, et al. Ledipasvir and sofosbuvir plus Ribavirin for treatment of HCV infection in patients with advanced liver disease. *Gastroenterology*. 2015;149:649–659.

6. Carrion AF, Khaderi SA, Sussman NL. Model for end-stage liver disease limbo, model for end-stage liver disease purgatory, and the dilemma of treating hepatitis C in patients awaiting liver transplantation. *Liver Transpl*. 2016;22:279–280.

7. Bhamidimarri KR, Ladino M, Pedraza F, et al. Transplantation of kidneys from hepatitis C-positive donors into hepatitis C virus-infected recipients followed by early initiation of direct acting antiviral therapy: a single-center retrospective study. *Transpl Int*. 2017;30:865–873.

8. Poordad F, Schiff ER, Vierling JM, et al. Daclatasvir with sofosbuvir and ribavirin for hepatitis C virus infection with advanced cirrhosis or post-liver transplantation recurrence. *Hepatology*. 2016;63:1493–1505.

9. Flemming JA, Kim WR, Brosgart CL, Terrault NA. Reduction in liver transplant wait-listing in the era of direct-acting antiviral therapy. *Hepatology*. 2017;65:804–812.

10. Martin P, Fabrizi F. Hepatitis C virus and kidney disease. *J Hepatol*. 2008;49:613–624.

11. Fabrizi F, Poordad FF, Martin P. Hepatitis C infection and the patient with end stage renal disease. *Hepatology*. 2002;36:3–10.

12. Fabrizi F, Martin P, Dixit V, Bunnapradist S, Dulai G. Meta-analysis: effect of hepatitis C virus infection on mortality in dialysis. *Aliment Pharmacol Ther*. 2004;20:1271–1277.

13. Hsu YC, Ho HJ, Huang YT, et al. Association between antiviral treatment and extrahepatic outcomes in patients with hepatitis C virus infection. *Gut*. 2015;64:495–503.

14. Fabrizi F, Martin P, Dixit V, Bunnapradist S, Dulai G. Hepatitis C virus antibody status and survival after renal transplantation: meta-analysis of observational studies. *Am J Transplant*. 2005;5:1452–1461.

15. Astor BC, Muntner P, Levin A, Eustace JA, Coresh J. Association of kidney function with anemia: the Third National Health and Nutrition Examination Survey (1988-1994). *Arch Intern Med*. 2002;162:1401–1408.

16. Nazario HE, Ndungu M, Modi AA. Sofosbuvir and simeprevir in hepatitis C genotype 1-patients with end-stage renal disease on haemodialysis or GFR <30 ml/min. *Liver Int*. 2016;36:798–801.

17. Bhamidimarri KR, Czul F, Peyton A, et al. Safety, efficacy and tolerability of half-dose sofosbuvir plus simeprevir in treatment of Hepatitis C in patients with end stage renal disease. *J Hepatol*. 2015;63:763–765.

18. Saxena V, Koraishy FM, Sise ME, et al. Safety and efficacy of sofosbuvir-containing regimens in hepatitis C-infected patients with impaired renal function. *Liver Int*. 2016;36:807–816.

19. Pockros PJ, Reddy KR, Mantry PS, et al. Efficacy of direct-acting antiviral combination for patients with hepatitis C virus genotype 1 infection and severe renal impairment or end-stage renal disease. *Gastroenterology*. 2016;150:1590–1598.

20. Roth D, Nelson DR, Bruchfeld A, et al. Grazoprevir plus elbasvir in treatment-naive and treatment-experienced patients with hepatitis C virus genotype 1 infection and stage 4-5 chronic kidney disease (the C-SURFER study): a combination phase 3 study. *Lancet*. 2015;386:1537–1545.

21. Gane E, Lawitz E, Pugatch D, et al. Glecaprevir and pibrentasvir in patients with HCV and severe renal impairement. *N Engl J Med*. 2017;377:1448–1455.

22. Rowe IA, Webb K, Gunson BK, Mehta N, Haque S, Neuberger J. The impact of disease recurrence on graft survival following liver transplantation: a single centre experience. *Transpl Int*. 2008;21:459–465.

23. Forman LM, Lewis JD, Berlin JA, Feldman HI, Lucey MR. The association between hepatitis C infection and survival after orthotopic liver transplantation. *Gastroenterology*. 2002;122:889–896.

24. Everson GT, Trotter J, Forman L, et al. Treatment of advanced hepatitis C with a low accelerating dosage regimen of antiviral therapy. *Hepatology*. 2005;42:255–262.

25. Faisal N, Bilodeau M, Aljudaibi B, et al. Sofosbuvir-based antiviral therapy is highly effective in recurrent hepatitis C in liver transplant recipients: Canadian multicenter "real-life" experience. *Transplantation*. 2016;100:1059–1065.

26. Leroy V, Dumortier J, Coilly A, et al. Efficacy of Sofosbuvir and daclatasvir in patients with fibrosing cholestatic hepatitis C after liver transplantation. *Clin Gastroenterol Hepatol*. 2015;13:1993–2001. e1991–1992.

27. Staples CT Jr., Rimland D, Dudas D. Hepatitis C in the HIV (human immunodeficiency virus) Atlanta VA (Veterans Affairs Medical Center) Cohort Study (HAVACS): the effect of coinfection on survival. *Clin Infect Dis*.1999;29:150–154.

28. Kim JH, Psevdos G, Suh J, Sharp VL. Co-infection of hepatitis B and hepatitis C virus in human immunodeficiency virus-infected patients in New York City, United States. *World J Gastroenterol*. 2008;14:6689–6693.

29. Spradling PR, Richardson JT, Buchacz K, et al. Trends in hepatitis C virus infection among patients in the HIV Outpatient Study, 1996–2007. *J Acquir Immune Defic Syndr*. 2010;53:388–396.

30. Thomas DL, Astemborski J, Rai RM, et al. The natural history of hepatitis C virus infection: host, viral, and environmental factors. *JAMA*. 2000;284:450–456.

31. Graham CS, Baden LR, Yu E, et al. Influence of human immunodeficiency virus infection on the course of hepatitis C virus infection: a meta-analysis. *Clin Infect Dis*. 2001;33:562–569.

32. Weber R, Sabin CA, Friis-Moller N, et al. Liver-related deaths in persons infected with the human immunodeficiency virus: the D:A:D study. *Arch Intern Med*. 2006;166:1632–1641.

33. Giordano TP, Kramer JR, Souchek J, Richardson P, El-Serag HB. Cirrhosis and hepatocellular carcinoma in HIV-infected veterans with and without the hepatitis C virus: a cohort study, 1992–2001. *Arch Intern Med*. 2004;164:2349–2354.

34. Matthews GV, Dore GJ. HIV and hepatitis C coinfection. *J Gastroenterol Hepatol*. 2008;23:1000–1008.

35. Berenguer J, Alvarez-Pellicer J, Martin PM, et al. Sustained virological response to interferon plus ribavirin reduces liver-related complications and mortality in patients coinfected with human immunodeficiency virus and hepatitis C virus. *Hepatology*. 2009;50:407–413.

36. Sulkowski MS, Naggie S, Lalezari J, et al. Sofosbuvir and ribavirin for hepatitis C in patients with HIV coinfection. *JAMA*. 2014;312:353–361.

37. Ghany MG, Strader DB, Thomas DL, Seeff LB, American Association for the Study of Liver D. Diagnosis, management, and treatment of hepatitis C: an update. *Hepatology*. 2009;49:1335–1374.

38. Costilla V, Mathur N, Gutierrez JA. Mechanisms of virologic failure with direct-acting antivirals in hepatitis C and strategies for retreatment. *Clin Liver Dis*. 2015;19:641–656.

39. Forns X, Gordon SC, Zuckerman E, et al. Grazoprevir and elbasvir plus ribavirin for chronic HCV genotype-1 infection after failure of combination therapy containing a direct-acting antiviral agent. *J Hepatol*. 2015;63:564–572.

40. Sulkowski M, Hezode C, Gerstoft J, et al. Efficacy and safety of 8 weeks versus 12 weeks of treatment with grazoprevir (MK-5172) and elbasvir (MK-8742) with or without ribavirin in patients with hepatitis C virus genotype 1 mono-infection and HIV/hepatitis C virus co-infection (C-WORTHY): a randomised, open-label phase 2 trial. *Lancet*. 2015;385:1087–1097.

41. Zeuzem S, Ghalib R, Reddy KR, et al. Grazoprevir-elbasvir combination therapy for treatment-naive cirrhotic and noncirrhotic patients with chronic hepatitis C virus genotype 1, 4, or 6 infection: a randomized trial. *Ann Intern Med*. 2015;163:1–13.

42. Sarrazin C. The importance of resistance to direct antiviral drugs in HCV infection in clinical practice. *J Hepatol*. 2015;64:486–504.

43. Kwo P, Gane EJ, Peng CY, et al. Effectiveness of elbasvir and grazoprevir combination, with or without ribavirin, for treatment-experienced patients with chronic hepatitis C infection. *Gastroenterology*. 2017;152:164–175 e164.

44. Bourliere M et al. Sofosbuvir, velpatasvir, and voxilaprevir for previously treated HCV infection. *N Engl J Med*. 2017;376:2134–2146.

45. Poordad F, et al. Glecaprevir and pibrentasvir for 12 weeks for hepatitis C virus genotype 1 infection and prior direct-acting antiviral treatment. *Hepatology*. 2017;66:389–397.

Chapter 12

Hepatitis C in Liver Transplantation

Justin R. Boike and Josh Levitsky

Introduction

Hepatitis C infection continues to be the leading indication worldwide for orthotopic liver transplantation (OLT).[1,2] All hepatitis C virus (HCV)-infected liver transplant recipients invariably develop recurrence, ranging from histologic evidence of mild inflammation to fibrosing cholestatic hepatitis (FCH), an accelerated form associated with extremely poor outcomes.[3–5] Combination oral direct-acting antivirals (DAA) have revolutionized the treatment of HCV both pre- and post-OLT, although further data are necessary to determine the optimal timing of treatment initiation.

Epidemiology and Risk Factors for Recurrence

The majority of OLT recipients develop histologic evidence of recurrence within 5 years of OLT. Within this group, 10–25% develop cirrhosis in the transplanted liver, while 2–9% develop FCH within 1 year.[6] Once HCV cirrhosis recurs, 40% of patients decompensate within 1 year, resulting in 1- and 4-year patient survival rates of 66% and 33%, respectively, highlighting the importance of developing an appropriate treatment plan either pre-, peri-, or posttransplant.

Risk factors for accelerated HCV recurrence are shown in Table 12.1.[7]

The best-identified risk factors for HCV recurrence with respect to the recipient relate to the level of immunosuppression in the peri- and postoperative period. Use of high-dosed intravenous corticosteroids at the time of induction or for the treatment of acute rejection has been associated with a near twofold increase in the rate of recurrence.[8] Data on the use of lympho-depleting antibodies such as antithymocyte globulin in the perioperative period are somewhat inconclusive.[9–11] Coinfection with HIV is risk factor for rapid recurrence and has been associated with 5-year overall survival of 50–60%.[12,13] Serological evidence of concomitant cytomegalovirus (CMV) infection has also been associated with a graft failure rate of 50% at 5 years compared to only 19% among CMV-negative recipients.[14] Interestingly, the

Table 12.1 Risk factors for accelerated HCV recurrence

Definite	Controversial	Not Clearly Associated
Acute rejection therapy: - Intravenous steroids - Lymphodepleting antibody	Corticosteroid therapy: - Use vs complete avoidance - Rapid vs slow tapering	Induction therapy: - IL-2 antibody - Lymphodepleting antibody
Recipient age	Viral load (>1 × 10⁶ copies/mL at transplant)	HCV + donor
Cytomegalovirus infection	Genotype 1b	Live donor
Ischemia/reperfusion injury	Donor after cardiac death	Maintenance immunosuppression
Diabetes mellitus	HLA mismatch	

severity of inflammation in the explanted liver correlates with the rate and severity of recurrence.[15]

Risk factors associated with the donor are also significant in predicting HCV recurrence. Due to the high demand for donor livers, various strategies have been implemented to expand the donor pool, including the use of marginal or expanded donor livers for transplantation. This includes using donors after cardiac death (DCD), donors older than 60 years of age, and HCV-infected donors. The impact on outcomes and recurrence in post-OLT HCV patients has been variable. Studies have shown that recipients of older donor livers (>60 years) and DCD livers (particularly from DCD donors who are older) have worse outcomes, including immediate perioperative complications and recurrent HCV-related cirrhosis/decompensation.[16,17] In DCD donors, HCV recurrence has been shown to be more rapid, but graft failure and patient survival rates do not appear to be affected. Data from the Organ Procurement and Transplant Network (OPTN) show that HCV-positive DCD recipients have 1- and 3-year patient survival rates of 84% and 75%, while HCV-negative DCD recipients have rates of 84% and 76%, respectively, suggesting no difference. The data for older donors are not as favorable. Both recurrence and patient survival are affected negatively by donor age of more than 60 years.[18–20] The mechanism by which older age is associated with poor outcomes is not well established but is likely multifactorial. Older-donor livers have a lower tolerance for preservation and a greater susceptibility to cold ischemia. Furthermore, age-related immune changes, such as liver steatosis, iron content, preexisting fibrosis, and changes in telomeres/senescence, may play a role in accelerating recurrence.[20] Historically, donors over 60 years of age were discouraged for HCV-positive recipients; however, this will likely change in the era of improved treatment options with oral DAAs. Donors after cardiac death younger than 60 years of age (and particularly <40) appear to have acceptable outcomes. HCV status of the donor has also been evaluated in predicting recurrence. Transplantation of HCV-infected grafts to HCV-infected recipients appears to have similar survival outcomes compared to HCV-negative donors.[21] Older donor age again contributes to a higher risk for more rapid advanced fibrosis in recipients.[22] Interestingly, recipients who retain their strain appear to have more severe liver disease.[20,23,24]

Other factors predisposing to increased risk that have no conclusive evidence include female gender, donor hypernatremia, prolonged hospitalization, African-American race, and pressor requirement perioperatively.[25]

Diagnosis

Monitoring of liver function tests (LFT) following OLT is done routinely, but abnormalities are common and do not differentiate between HCV recurrence and other etiologies of LFT abnormalities, particularly allograft rejection. The gold standard for diagnosing HCV recurrence versus rejection is liver biopsy. However, despite being the gold standard, histologic evaluation of the allograft is often not specific enough to differentiate between recurrence and early graft rejection.[26]

To evaluate for acute rejection, pathologists rely on the Banff criteria, looking for the presence of a mixed portal inflammatory infiltrate composed of lymphocytes, eosinophils, and neutrophils, along with ductilitis and endothelitis with minimal hepatocyte damage (Figure 12.1). In chronic rejection, there is loss of intrahepatic/interlobular bile ducts, subintimal fibrosis, and foam cell changes in large- and medium-caliber hilar hepatic arteries and portal veins (Figure 12.2). Due to technical limitations, the diagnostic vascular changes are rarely present in needle biopsy specimens.

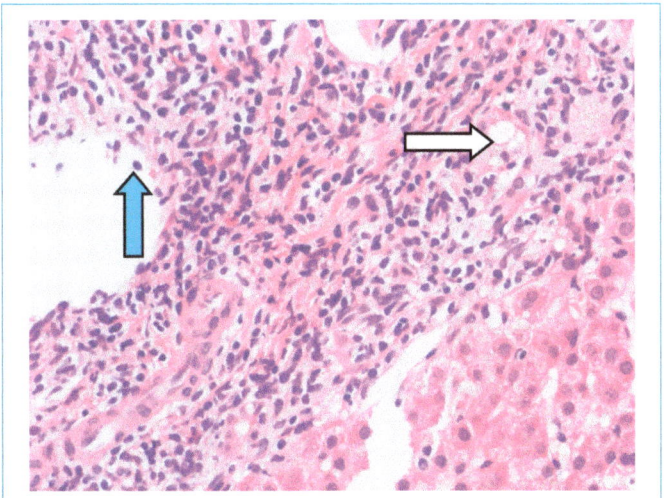

Figure 12.1 Acute cellular rejection. Portal tract with mixed inflammatory infiltrate composed of lymphocytes, neutrophils, and eosinophils. There is damage to the bile ducts (*white arrow*) and undermining/sloughing of the venous endothelium (*blue arrow*)

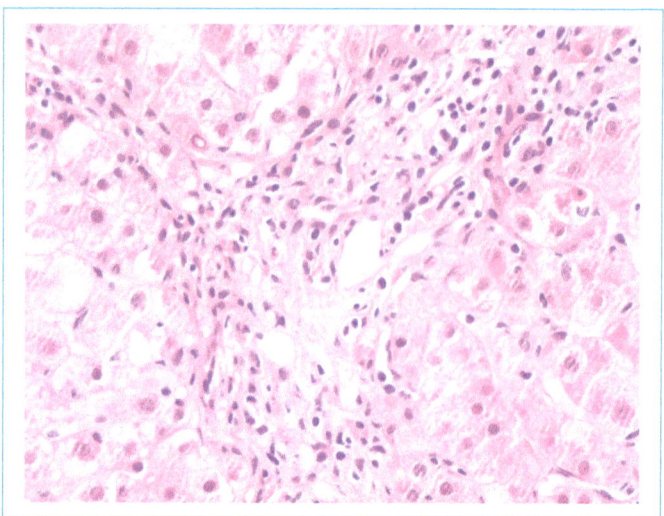

Figure 12.2 Chronic ductopenic rejection. This portal tract demonstrates the loss of an intrahepatic/interlobular bile duct with minimal portal inflammation

Histologic features of HCV recurrence in the liver allograft are similar to those in a nontransplanted liver and can present as early, established, or progressive changes. In the early phase, there is mild, nonspecific portal inflammation. An established infection presents as acute hepatitis approximately 2–4 months posttransplantation. The histologic findings include lobular hepatocyte disarray, ballooning change, and Mallory bodies (Figure 12.3). With progressive chronic infection, there is a predominantly portal infiltrate composed of lymphocytes often with lymphoid follicle formation, the presence of occasional plasma cells and/or eosinophils, and mild macrovesicular fatty change with minimal acidophil bodies (Figure 12.4). When compared to the nontransplanted patient, the course of HCV is often more aggressive, with recurrence in the allograft as demonstrated by more severe inflammatory activity and rapid progression to fibrosis, with a 5-year risk of cirrhosis ranging from 8% to 28%. Certain features in early posttransplant biopsies may suggest a more rapid progression to fibrosis and include severity of necroinflammatory activity, presence and severity of macrovesicular steatosis in day 1 to 28 liver biopsies, and presence of prominent hepatocyte ballooning and cholestasis (Samuel, Forns et al. 2006).[24]

Historically, additional stratification for evidence of advanced fibrosis was necessary to determine who was an appropriate candidate to treat with interferon (IFN)-based HCV therapies that had multiple side effects and were difficult to tolerate. Considering the availability, safety, and tolerability of oral DAAs, all patients with HCV recurrence should be recommended for treatment, thus essentially eliminating the need for risk stratification by biopsy. Countries with limited access or restrictions to DAA therapy, however, may still rely on serial liver biopsies for evidence of HCV recurrence, along with other assessments

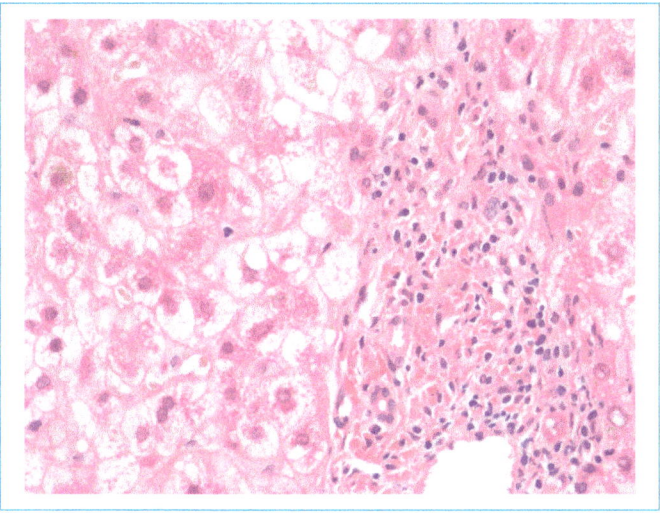

Figure 12.3 Acute hepatitis C recurrence. The lobule is notable for hepatocyte disarray, ballooning change, and the presence of Mallory bodies. Within the portal tract, there is minimal inflammation composed of lymphocytes and plasma cells. No evidence of acute rejection is seen

of fibrosis to determine treatment candidates. Fibrosis assessments include invasive measurement of the hepatic venous pressure gradient (HVPG) and noninvasive measurement of liver stiffness. An elevated HVPG (>10 mm Hg) suggests development of portal hypertension and has been shown to predict progression to more advanced disease.[27,28] Liver stiffness, as measured by transient elastography or magnetic resonance imaging (MRI) elastography offers a noninvasive measure of fibrosis and has a higher sensitivity and positive predictive value for advanced fibrosis compared to other clinical markers.[29,30]

Treatment

Historically, the IFN-based therapies for HCV were associated with a significant toxicity profile and posed a risk of hepatic decompensation to those with cirrhosis awaiting OLT. Similarly, posttransplant HCV was difficult to treat due to high rates of treatment failure and premature discontinuation from multisystem adverse effects, such as flu-like illness, cytopenia, psychiatric, neurologic, and the like. Hence, the window for HCV treatment before and after OLT was limited. The paradigm for HCV treatment in the transplant population has shifted dramatically with the development of oral DAAs. In the pretransplant setting, for those with decompensated cirrhosis, there is a potential to reverse fibrosis and decompensation through achievement of SVR.[31] In those who are destined for transplantation, the goals of treatment are to suppress viral loads to undetectable levels in order to prevent graft

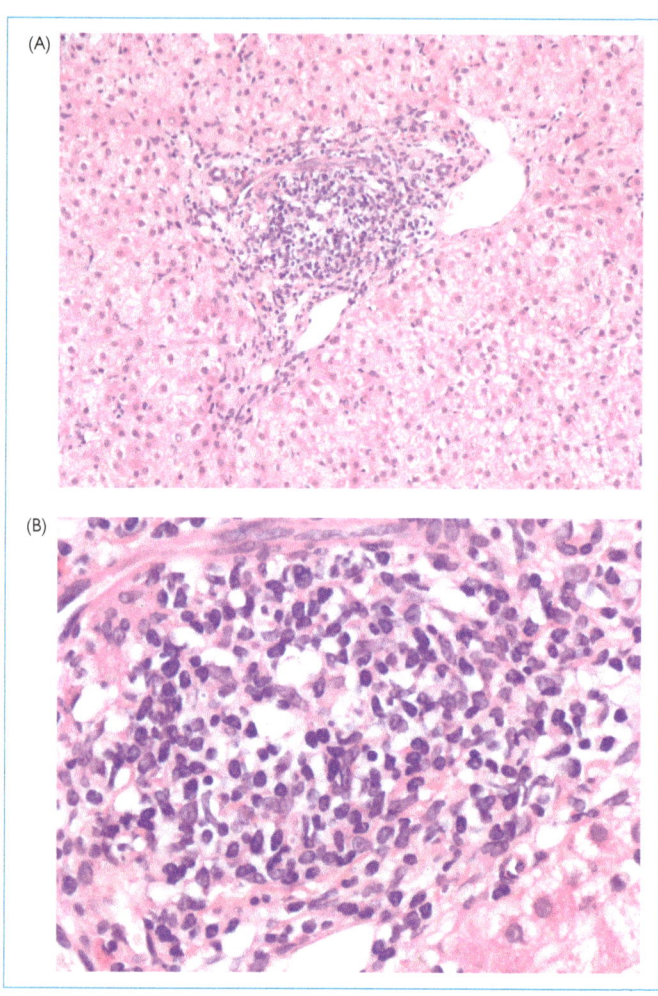

Figure 12.4 Recurrent hepatitis C. (A) Predominantly portal inflammatory infiltrate with minimal lobular activity. (B) Lymphoid follicle formation composed of lymphocytes with an occasional plasma cell

reinfection and histological recurrence. Finally, in the posttransplant setting, treating established HCV recurrence or before it occurs can prevent fibrosis progression and limit the need for retransplantation.

Pretransplant

A viral load greater than 1×10^6 copies/mL at transplant is associated with a higher risk of rapid HCV recurrence. Clearance of HCV viremia resulting in SVR prior to OLT is beneficial for multiple reasons including reduced rates of all-cause mortality, hepatic decompensation, hepatocellular carcinoma (HCC), and a reduced risk of recurrence post-OLT.[32–36] With the emergence of oral combination DAA therapies, higher rates of SVR (>95%) can now be achieved without the risks of toxicity and hepatic decompensation as per previous IFN-based therapies. The field of HCV treatment is rapidly changing, and the reader is encouraged to visit www.hcvguidelines.org for comprehensive, real-time recommendations of available HCV treatments as per a joint effort by the American Association for the Study of Liver Disease (AASLD) and Infectious Diseases Society of America (IDSA). Patient factors that should be considered prior to initiation of treatment in the pretransplant setting include renal function, cirrhosis (compensated vs. decompensated), and prior treatment experience. In general, decompensated cirrhosis, defined by Child-Turcotte-Pugh (CTP) Class B or C, often requires concomitant administration of weight-based ribavirin (RBV) and is associated with lower rates of SVR (83–87%) compared to rates of greater than 97% in compensated cirrhosis (CTP Class A).[37,38] While there are no prospective data, modeling studies have suggested that treatment in the pretransplant stage is most clinically and cost effective for individuals with model for end-stage liver (MELD) scores of less than 25, and those with higher MELD scores should probably be treated after OLT.[39] This still remains an area of significant debate, and further study is warranted to determine the ideal timing of treatment.[40]

In patients with compensated cirrhosis with concomitant HCC who need OLT, regardless of the treatment regimen chosen, the goal of treatment should be to clear the virus from the bloodstream prior to transplantation. Patients who have obtained SVR, however, are generally not candidates for HCV-infected donor organs, and this may limit their access to some portion of the donor pool.[7] In most instances, waitlist times vary, and, as such, it can be difficult to predict when OLT will occur. There are limited data surrounding treatment strategies that intersect with OLT. A phase 2, open label study investigating the effect of 48 weeks of sofosbuvir (SOF) and RBV among those with compensated cirrhosis on the waitlist for HCC demonstrated that an undetectable viral load for longer than 28 days prior to OLT conferred a post-OLT SVR rate of 95% (23/24). Conversely, those who had detectable levels of viral load less than 28 days prior to OLT (9/10) developed HCV recurrence after OLT.[41] This suggests that if treatment is employed among those awaiting OLT, then the goal should be achievement of virologic clearance at least 28 days prior to transplant.

Some have hypothesized that treatment of HCV may modulate HCC tumor biology or prevent recurrence in patients who are not OLT candidates.[42] Unfortunately, recent prospective reports have not demonstrated a reduction in the rates of recurrent HCC among those patients who achieve SVR.[43]

Among patients with decompensated cirrhosis, treatment data with combination DAAs are less robust, with some promising results. SVR rates of as high as 86% can be achieved even in CTP Class C patients with regimens including ledipasivir + sofosbuvir (LDV + SOF), sofosbuvir + velpatasvir (SOF + VEL), or daclatasvir + sofosbuvir (DCV + SOF), all with or without RBV.[37,44–46] Previous use of first-generation protease inhibitors, including boceprevir and telaprevir, was associated with further liver decompensation in patients with advanced liver disease. Hence the use of newer generations of protease inhibitors, including simeprevir, is discouraged in those with decompensated cirrhosis. Successful treatment of HCV in decompensated cirrhosis can lead to improved biochemical parameters as well as improved clinical outcomes, including ascites and hepatic encephalopathy,[44] more typically in lower (<20) MELD patients. There is significant debate in the field in terms of treating decompensated transplant candidates as this could potentially "lower" their position on the waitlist due to improvements of their native MELD scores, with questionable clinical improvement.[45] Presently, there is limited evidence to support this claim. Among the studies treating HCV in decompensated cirrhosis, very few patients with MELD scores of greater than 20 were included, limiting the ability to make firm conclusions regarding treatment in this population.[37,44,46–48] However, it appears reasonable to treat patients with MELD scores of less than 20 with the goal of either attaining a compensated state and avoiding the need for OLT or eradicating the virus before transplantation if liver transplant is inevitable or required.

Perioperative

There are limited data regarding the treatment of HCV at the time of OLT. Attempts have included infusion of human monoclonal antibody targeting the HCV E2 glycoprotein (MBL-HCV1) at the time of transplant to limit the post-OLT viremia.[49] While this was associated with a delay in recurrent viremia, subjects had resistance-associated variants at the time of viral rebound. A further study combining MBL-HCV1 with a single-agent oral DAA was underpowered, with eight patients receiving telaprevir (which is no longer recommended) and only two receiving sofosbuvir.[50] More promising data are from an open label, phase 2 study in which LDV + SOF treatment was initiated on the day of OLT followed by continuation for 4 weeks. Sustained virologic response was achieved in 14/16 (88%), and one of the treatment failures was associated with baseline resistance mutations. The patient with resistance was subsequently treated with an additional 12 weeks of therapy and achieved SVR, yielding an overall SVR rate of 15/16 (94%) post-OLT.[51] This suggests that, in patients who cannot be treated prior to transplantation, treatment with DAA therapy at the time of transplantation may be a safe, cost-effective approach.

Posttransplant

In the era of IFN-based therapies, recommendations were to monitor the patient with serial liver biopsies and initiate treatment only at the time of histological recurrence given the toxicity of treatments.[52] The paradigm of treatment has shifted, and now the recommendation is to treat all patients with HCV viremia recurrence after OLT, regardless of histological evidence of recurrence. The goals of HCV treatment in the posttransplant setting include achievement of SVR as well as minimizing the risk of developing HCV-associated complications such as graft failure, hepatic fibrosis, and FCH. Furthermore, the treatment of HCV with achievement of SVR is associated with improved graft function and patient survival.[20] The timing of when to initiate treatment after OLT, however, remains unknown. Enrollment criteria for clinical trials of DAAs in the post-OLT setting generally required at least

3 months from transplant, and often patients were several years out from transplant. Factors that influence timing of therapy mainly involve renal function and potential drug–drug interactions with immunosuppression. There can be significant fluctuations in renal function immediately post-OLT, and this often requires close monitoring and adjustment of immunosuppression dosing, specifically calcineurin inhibitors (Table 12.2).

Given that most post-OLT treatment regimens rely on RBV, which is dosed based on renal function, consensus is to await stabilization of renal function prior to initiation of a treatment plan. For those with normal renal function, current AASLD-IDSA recommendations are to treat recurrent HCV infection of genotypes 1 and 4 in OLT recipients, including compensated cirrhosis, with a 12-week course of LDV + SOF in combination with weight dosed RBV.[53]

Ledipasvir and SOF have no significant drug interactions with immunosuppressive regimens. SVR rates at 12 weeks with LDV + SOF and RBV were 96–98% for noncirrhotic patients and 60–96% for those with cirrhosis.[37] SVR rates are lower among those with more severe liver disease defined by higher CTP Class B/C. Current recommendations are to treat those with decompensated cirrhosis, CTP Class B/C, with 12-weeks of LDV + SOF with low-dose initial RBV (600 mg) and to increase RBV as tolerated.[54]

Table 12.2 Oral direct-acting antivirals (DAAs) and interactions with calcineurin inhibitors

DAA	Cyclosporine (CSA)	Tacrolimus (TAC)
Sofosbuvir (SOF)	Monitor CSA levels and titrate CSA dose as needed	Monitor TAC levels and titrate TAC dose as needed
Ledipasvir (LDV)	Monitor CSA levels and titrate CSA dose as needed	Monitor TAC levels and titrate TAC dose as needed
Daclatasvir (DCL)	Monitor CSA levels and titrate CSA dose as needed	Monitor TAC levels and titrate TAC dose as needed
Simeprevir (SIM)	↑ in SIM; combination is not recommended	Monitor TAC levels and titrate TAC dose as needed
Paritaprevir + ritonavir + ombitasvir + dasabuvir(PrOD)	↑ in CSA; modeling suggest using 1/5 of CSA dose during PrOD treatment, monitor CSA levels and titrate CSA dose as needed	↑↑↑ in TAC; modeling suggests TAC 0.5 mg every 7 days during PrOD treatment, monitor TAC levels and titrate TAC dose as needed
Elbasvir/Grazoprevir (EBR/GZR)	↑↑ in GZR AUC and ↑ in EBR AUC; combination is not recommended	↑↑ in TAC; monitor TAC levels and titrate TAC dose as needed
Velpatasvir	Monitor CSA levels and titrate CSA dose as needed	Monitor TAC levels and titrate TAC dose as needed

Adapted from www.hcvguidelines.org (AASLD-IDSA).

If RBV is contraindicated, then therapy with LDV + SOF should be extended to 24 weeks. Alternative regimens include fixed-dosed paritaprevir-ritonavir-ombitasvir with dasabuvir (PrOD) along with weight-dosed RBV among OLT recipients with early fibrosis. This regimen, however, is associated with significantly increased trough levels of calcineurin inhibitors requiring prospective dosing modifications.[55] For genotypes 2 and 3, treatment recommendations include daclatasvir-sofosbuvir (DCV + SOF) along with low-dose RBV for 12 weeks and extension to 24 weeks in those in whom RBV is contraindicated.

Patients with advanced chronic kidney disease and those requiring dialysis have been challenging to treat due to the inability to use a SOF-containing regimen. Elbasvir and grazoprevir (EBR + GZR), however, is approved and has SVR rates of 90% in patients with advanced renal insufficiency and those requiring dialysis.[56] It has not, however, been studied among the OLT population, and there are likely significant drug–drug interactions with the calcineurin inhibitors.

There are no prospective treatment data for those who have the presence of a mixed infection of more than one genotype among OLT patients with HCV recurrence. Expert consensus is to treat with a regimen that maximizes efficacy against both genotypes. Pan-genotypic regimens such as sofosbuvir-velpatasvir (SOF + VEL) have recently been approved, although this has yet to be studied in the post-OLT population.[46,57]

Retransplantation

The decision to relist a patient with recurrent HCV cirrhosis post-OLT is made on a case-by-case basis and remains a controversial issue among transplant centers. Retransplantation for all indications generally has a poorer prognosis, with 3-year survival rates of approximately 49% among HCV recurrence compared to 55% in non-HCV patients.[58,59] Furthermore, the severity and rapidity of HCV recurrence and fibrosis are often similar or worse in nature to the initial graft recurrence. New DAA therapies have again shifted this paradigm, and treatment of HCV prior to or right after retransplantation will likely improve outcomes and further reduce the need for retransplantation. Data in this realm are limited to case reports, and no prospective trials or practice guidelines are yet available to guide providers.[60]

Fibrosing Cholestatic Hepatitis

FCH is a rare but severe form of recurrent HCV that until recently portended a grim prognosis for recipients. It is characterized by severe cholestatic injury and rapidly progressive liver dysfunction that occurs generally within weeks of liver transplantation in approximately 5–10% of HCV-positive recipients. The first histologic account in the literature described a pattern of "extensive dense portal fibrosis with immature fibrous bands extending into sinusoidal spaces, ductal proliferation and hypercellularity, marked canalicular and cellular cholestasis, and moderate mononuclear inflammation" (Figure 12.5).[61] Today, distinguishing FCH from other forms of hepatitis or graft injury remains a challenge and cannot rely solely on histologic interpretation, but rather

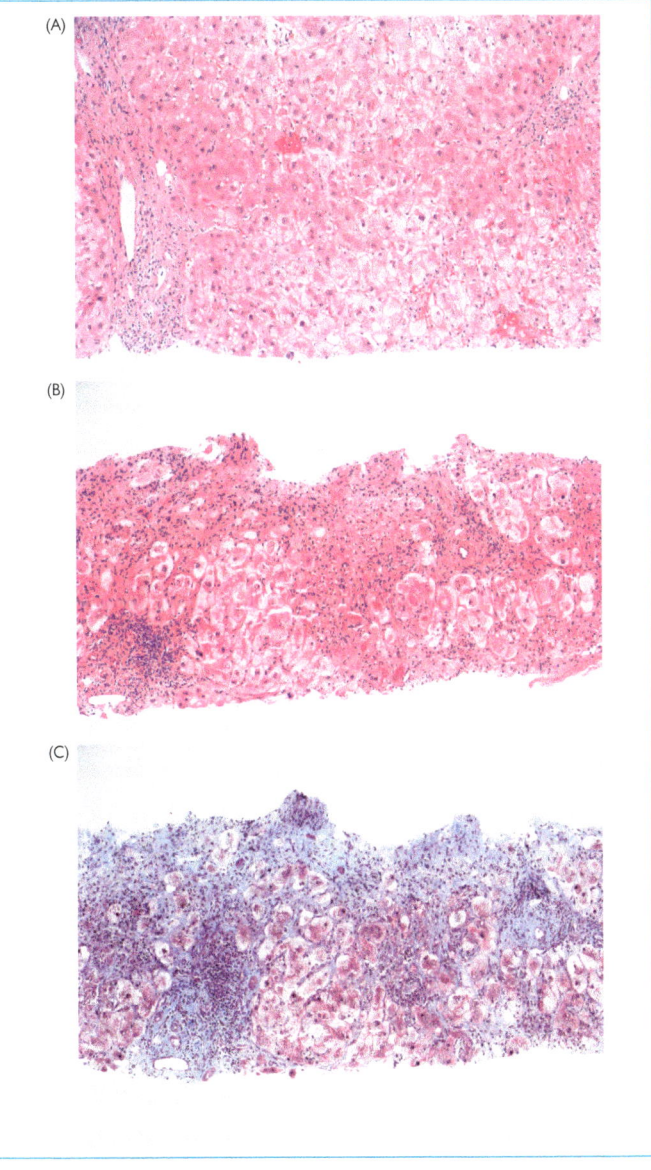

Figure 12.5 Fibrosing cholestatic hepatitis. (A) Biopsy 15 months posttransplant demonstrates mild portal inflammation, diffuse ballooning change, and mild cholestasis. (B) Biopsy 5 months later (20 months posttransplant) reveals cirrhosis. (C) Confirmation of cirrhosis using Masson's trichrome stain to highlight fibrosis and demonstrated by the blue staining

combines clinical, biochemical, and serologic profiles. Historically, most cases were fatal despite attempts at treatment and changes in immunosuppression.

Unfortunately, it is difficult to predict who will develop FCH as there are no clear risk factors other than the use of high-dose intravenous corticosteroids or lympho-depleting immunosuppressive agents. Genotype, type of immunosuppression, HCV viral load, and combined liver-kidney transplantation have also been suggested as risk factors, but the data on these have been equivocal. The pathogenesis for FCH is poorly understood, but a proposed mechanism involves hepatocyte repopulation and regeneration after liver transplantation.[62] Injury of hepatocytes is thought to be from a direct cytopathic effect of HCV as there is a relative absence of inflammation, a high serum viral load, and many HCV virions in the hepatocytes. After transplantation, within hours of graft reperfusion, viral loads return to pretransplant levels, and significantly high levels of viremia can lead to the rapid cytopathic effect seen in FCH. Interestingly, studies have shown that patients with mild recurrent HCV have more genetic diversification in their genomic RNA viral sequences than do patients who develop FCH, suggesting that homogeneity in the viral sequences post-OLT may predispose to FCH.

One important challenge when reviewing post-OLT complications is to distinguish FCH or aggressive recurrence from acute cellular rejection. Some histologic clues can aid in differentiating the two. In FCH, the earliest changes are typically lobular without affecting the portal regions, such as those seen in acute cellular rejection, including endothelitis, ductilitis, and mixed portal-inflammatory infiltrates. The initial changes in FCH include centrilobular (zone 3) hepatocyte ballooning degeneration with mild inflammatory activity. The degree of cholestasis can vary at this stage. As the disease progresses, portal changes become more prominent, and bile ductular proliferation and portal expansion due to the inflammatory infiltrate occurs. The degree of fibrosis then progresses from pericellular and perisinusoidal to bridging fibrosis and, in some cases, to cirrhosis. Chronic graft rejection can also lead to cholestasis and may be hard to distinguish from FCH. In the former, foam cell changes and a lack of intrahepatic/interlobular bile ducts are prominent (see Figure 12.1), which are not typical of FCH. New diagnostic criteria have been proposed that combine histological findings along with laboratory parameters such as bilirubin and donor characteristics.[63] As escalation of immunosuppression can be devastating for a patient with FCH, it is imperative to distinguish it from acute cellular rejection as clearly as possible, using viral load (usually extremely high in FCH) and biochemical, clinical, and histological pieces of evidence.

Fortunately, FCH is now a treatable condition, and SVR is attainable with oral DAA therapies. Several clinical trials evaluating the efficacy of combination DAAs in HCV recurrence among post-OLT patients also enrolled cases of FCH. The results were just as promising with combinations of SOF + SIM with RBV for 24 weeks achieving 12-week SVR in 13/13 (100%) of cases meeting criteria for FCH.[64] Similar results of 100% (6/6) SVR were obtained from a combination of LDV + SOF with RBV for 12–24 weeks duration.[37] Others looking at SOF + DCV and SOF + RBV demonstrated SVR in 22/23 (96%) after 24 weeks of therapy with 100% survival.[65] While FCH remains a possible complication of recurrent HCV, combination DAA therapies now can achieve impressive rates of viral clearance, rendering FCH much less of a threat to graft survival.

Conclusion

Hepatitis C recurrence is universal in patients undergoing OLT, and, historically, a significant percentage developed cirrhosis and complications within 5 years of transplantation. Treatment of HCV has been revolutionized with combination oral DAAs. SVR rates of nearly 100% can be achieved in patients even with compensated cirrhosis. Treatment of HCV in the decompensated cirrhotic patient remains challenging, raising the question of whether treatment should be deferred until the time of or after OLT in those who are candidates. Currently, there is evidence that achieving undetectable viral levels at least 4 weeks prior to OLT can prevent HCV recurrence in the graft. Other data suggest that initiation of DAAs on the day of transplant can achieve SVR with just 4 weeks of treatment. For those with HCV recurrence post-OLT, prospective studies have demonstrated similar rates of SVR to the pre-OLT population. These data have also demonstrated safety and tolerability without significant adjustments in immunosuppression. FCH, a once dreaded complication of HCV recurrence, can now be successfully treated, with improvement in graft function and survival.

References

1. Verna EC, Brown RS. Hepatitis C virus and liver transplantation. *Clin Liver Dis.* 2006;10(4):91–940.
2. Kim, WR, Stock, PG, Smith, JM, et al. OPTN/SRTR 2011 annual data report: liver. *Am J Transplant.* 2013;13(s1):73–102.
3. Greenberg HB. Recurrent and acquired hepatitis C viral infection in liver transplant recipients. *Gastroenterology.* 1992;103(1):317–322.
4. Berenguer M. Natural history of recurrent hepatitis C. *Liver Transplant.* 2002;8(10B):S14–S18.
5. Satapathy SK, Sclair S, Fiel MI, et al. Clinical characterization of patients developing histologically-proven fibrosing cholestatic hepatitis C post-liver transplantation. *Hepatol Res.* 2011;41(4):328–339.
6. Berenguer M, Schuppan D. Progression of liver fibrosis in post-transplant hepatitis C: mechanisms, assessment and treatment. *J Hepatol.* 2013;58(5):1028–1041.
7. Levitsky J, Doucette K. Viral hepatitis in solid organ transplantation. *Am J Transplant.* 2013;13(s4):147–168.
8. Charlton M, Seaberg E, Wiesner R, et al. Predictors of patient and graft survival following liver transplantation for hepatitis C. *Hepatology.* 1998;28(3):823–830.
9. Eason JD, Nair S, Cohen AJ, et al. Steroid-free liver transplantation using rabbit antithymocyte globulin and early tacrolimus monotherapy1. *Transplantation.* 2003;75(8):1396–1399.
10. De Ruvo N, Cucchetti A, Lauro A, et al. Preliminary results of a 'proper' tolerogenic regimen with thymoglobulin pretreatment and hepatitis C virus recurrence in liver transplantation. *Transplantation.* 2005;80(1):8–12.

11. Nair S, Loss GE, Cohen AJ, et al. Induction with rabbit antithymocyte globulin versus induction with corticosteroids in liver transplantation: impact on recurrent hepatitis C virus infection. *Transplantation.* 2006;81(4):620–622.

12. Ragni MV, Belle SH. Impact of human immunodeficiency virus infection on progression to end-stage liver disease in individuals with hemophilia and hepatitis C virus infection. *J Infect Dis.* 2001;183(7):1112–1115.

13. Eguchi S, Takatsuki M, Kuroki T. Liver transplantation for patients with human immunodeficiency virus and hepatitis C virus co-infection: update in 2013. *J Hepato-Biliar-Pancreatic Sci.* 2014;21(4):263–268.

14. Burak KW, Kremers WK, Batts KP, et al. Impact of cytomegalovirus infection, year of transplantation, and donor age on outcomes after liver transplantation for hepatitis C. *Liver Transplant.* 2002;8(4):362–369.

15. Ghabril M, Dickson RC, Krishna M, et al. Explanted liver inflammatory grade predicts fibrosis progression in hepatitis C recurrence. *Liver Transplant.* 2011;17(6):685–694.

16. Alonso O, Loinaz C, Moreno E, et al. Advanced donor age increases the risk of severe recurrent hepatitis C after liver transplantation. *Transplant Int.* 2005;18(8):902–907.

17. Yagci G, Fernandez LA, Knechtle SJ, et al. *The impact of donor variables on the outcome of orthotopic liver transplantation for hepatitis C.* Transplantation proceedings. Philadelphia: Elsevier; 2008.

18. Berenguer M, Prieto M, Juan FS, et al. Contribution of donor age to the recent decrease in patient survival among HCV-infected liver transplant recipients. *Hepatology.* 2002;36(1):202–210.

19. Lake JR, Shorr JS, Steffen BJ, et al. Differential effects of donor age in liver transplant recipients infected with hepatitis B, hepatitis C and without viral hepatitis. *Am J Transplant.* 2005;5(3):549–557.

20. Berenguer M. Risk of extended criteria donors in hepatitis c virus–positive recipients. *Liver Transplant.* 2008;14:S45–S50.

21. Vargas HE, Laskus T, Wang LF, et al. Outcome of liver transplantation in hepatitis C virus–infected patients who received hepatitis C virus–infected grafts. *Gastroenterology.* 1999;117(1):149–153.

22. Lai JC, O'leary JG, Trotter JF, et al. Risk of advanced fibrosis with grafts from hepatitis C antibody–positive donors: a multicenter cohort study. *Liver Transplant.* 2012;18(5):532–538.

23. Velidedeoglu E, Desai NM, Campos L, et al. The outcome of liver grafts procured from hepatitis C-positive donors. *Transplantation.* 2002;73(4):582–587.

24. Samuel D, Forns X, Berenguer M, et al. Report of the Monothematic EASL Conference on Liver Transplantation for Viral Hepatitis:(Paris, France, January 12–14, 2006). *J Hepatol.* 2006;45(1):127–143.

25. Feng S, Goodrich NP, Bragg-Gresham JL, et al. Characteristics associated with liver graft failure: the concept of a donor risk index. *Am J Transplant.* 2006;6(4):783–790.

26. Skripenova S, Trainer TD, Krawitt EL, et al. Variability of grade and stage in simultaneous paired liver biopsies in patients with hepatitis C. *J Clin Pathol.* 2007;60(3):321–324.

27. Blasco A, Forns X, Carrión JA, et al. Hepatic venous pressure gradient identifies patients at risk of severe hepatitis C recurrence after liver transplantation. *Hepatology.* 2006;43(3):492–499.

28. Kalambokis G, Manousou P, Samonakis D, et al. Clinical outcome of HCV-related graft cirrhosis and prognostic value of hepatic venous pressure gradient. *Transplant Int.* 2009;22(2):172–181.

29. Carrión JA, Navasa M, Bosch J, et al. Transient elastography for diagnosis of advanced fibrosis and portal hypertension in patients with hepatitis C recurrence after liver transplantation. *Liver Transplant.* 2006;12(12):1791–1798.

30. Lee VS, Miller FH, Omary RA, et al. Magnetic resonance elastography and biomarkers to assess fibrosis from recurrent hepatitis C in liver transplant recipients. *Transplantation.* 2011;92(5):581–586.

31. Cheung MC, Walker AJ, Hudson BE, et al. Outcomes after successful direct-acting antiviral therapy for patients with chronic hepatitis C and decompensated cirrhosis. *J Hepatol.* 2016;65(4):741–747.

32. Forman LM, Lewis JD, Berlin JA, et al. The association between hepatitis C infection and survival after orthotopic liver transplantation. *Gastroenterology.* 2002;122(4):889–896.

33. Veldt BJ, Heathcote EJ, Wedemeyer H, et al. Sustained virologic response and clinical outcomes in patients with chronic hepatitis C and advanced fibrosis. *Ann Intern Med.* 2007;147(10):677–684.

34. van der Meer AJ, Veldt BJ, Feld JJ, et al. Association between sustained virological response and all-cause mortality among patients with chronic hepatitis C and advanced hepatic fibrosis. *JAMA.* 2012;308(24):2584–2593.

35. van der Meer AJ, Wedemeyer H, Feld JJ, et al. Life expectancy in patients with chronic HCV infection and cirrhosis compared with a general population. *JAMA.* 2014;312(18):1927–1928.

36. Fortune BE, Martinez-Camacho A, Kreidler S, et al. Post-transplant survival is improved for hepatitis C recipients who are RNA negative at time of liver transplantation. *Transplant Int.* 2015;28(8):980–989.

37. Charlton M, Everson GT, Flamm SL, et al. Ledipasvir and sofosbuvir plus ribavirin for treatment of HCV infection in patients with advanced liver disease. *Gastroenterology.* 2015;149(3):649–659.

38. Gane EJ, Hyland RH, An D, et al. Efficacy of ledipasvir and sofosbuvir, with or without ribavirin, for 12 weeks in patients with HCV genotype 3 or 6 infection. *Gastroenterology.* 2015;149(6):1454–1461. e1451.

39. Njei B, McCarty TR, Fortune BE, et al. Optimal timing for hepatitis C therapy in US patients eligible for liver transplantation: a cost-effectiveness analysis. *Alimentary Pharmacol Therapeutics.* 2016;44(10):1090–1101.

40. Gallegos-Orozco JF, Charlton MR Treatment of HCV prior to liver transplantation to prevent HCV recurrence–Wise or wasteful? *Liver Int.* 2015;35(1):9–11.

41. Curry MP, Forns X, Chung RT, et al. Sofosbuvir and ribavirin prevent recurrence of HCV infection after liver transplantation: an open-label study. *Gastroenterology.* 2015;148(1):100–107. e101.

42. Hoshida Y, Fuchs BC, Bardeesy N, et al. Pathogenesis and prevention of hepatitis C virus-induced hepatocellular carcinoma. *J Hepatol.* 2014;61(1): S79–S90.

43. Conti F, Buonfiglioli F, Scuteri A, et al. Early occurrence and recurrence of hepatocellular carcinoma in HCV-related cirrhosis treated with direct-acting antivirals. *J Hepatol.* 2016;65(4):727–733.

44. Afdhal N, Everson G, Calleja JL, et al. O68 sofosbuvir and ribavirin for the treatment of chronic HCV with cirrhosis and portal hypertension with and without decompensation: early virologic response and safety. *J Hepatol.* 2014;60(1):S28.

45. Carrion AF, Khaderi SA, Sussman NL. Model for end-stage liver disease limbo, model for end-stage liver disease purgatory, and the dilemma of treating hepatitis C in patients awaiting liver transplantation. *Liver Transplant.* 2016;22(3):279–280.

46. Curry MP, O'Leary JG, Bzowej N, et al. Sofosbuvir and velpatasvir for HCV in patients with decompensated cirrhosis. *N Engl J Med.* 2015;373(27):2618–2628.

47. Modi AA, Nazario H, Trotter JF, et al. Safety and efficacy of Simeprevir plus Sofosbuvir with or without Ribavirin in patients with decompensated genotype 1 hepatitis C cirrhosis. *Liver Transplant.* 2016 Mar 1;22(3):281–286.

48. Poordad F, Schiff ER, Vierling JM, et al. Daclatasvir with sofosbuvir and ribavirin for hepatitis C virus infection with advanced cirrhosis or post-liver transplantation recurrence. *Hepatology.* 2016 May 1;63(5):1493–1505.

49. Chung RT, Gordon FD, Curry MP, et al. Human monoclonal antibody MBL-HCV1 delays HCV viral rebound following liver transplantation: a randomized controlled study. *Am J Transplant.* 2013;13(4):1047–1054.

50. Smith HL, Chung RT, Mantry P, et al. Prevention of allograft HCV recurrence with peri-transplant human monoclonal antibody MBL-HCV1 combined with a single oral direct-acting antiviral: a proof-of-concept study. *J Viral Hepatitis.* 2017 Mar 1;24(3):197–206.

51. Levitsky J, Verna EC, O'Leary JG, et al. Perioperative ledipasvir–sofosbuvir for HCV in liver-transplant recipients. *N Engl J Med.* 2016;375(21):2106–2108.

52. Chalasani N, Manzarbeitia C, Ferenci P, et al. Peginterferon alfa-2a for hepatitis C after liver transplantation: two randomized, controlled trials. *Hepatology.* 2005;41(2):289–298.

53. AASLD-IDSA. Recommendations for testing, managing, and treating hepatitis C. Retrieved January 17, 2017, from http://www.hcvguidelines.org/.

54. Reddy RK, Everson GT, Flamm SL, et al. Ledipasvir/sofosbuvir with ribavirin for the treatment of HCV in patients with post transplant recurrence: preliminary results of a prospective, multicenter study. *Hepatology.* 2014;60:200A–201A.

55. Kwo PY, Mantry PS, Coakley E, et al. An interferon-free antiviral regimen for HCV after liver transplantation. *N Engl J Med.* 2014;371(25):2375–2382.

56. Roth D, Nelson DR, Bruchfeld A, et al. Grazoprevir plus elbasvir in treatment-naive and treatment-experienced patients with hepatitis C virus genotype 1 infection and stage 4–5 chronic kidney disease (the C-SURFER study): a combination phase 3 study. *Lancet.* 2015;386(10003):1537–1545.

57. Feld JJ, Jacobson IM, Hézode C, et al. Sofosbuvir and velpatasvir for HCV genotype 1, 2, 4, 5, and 6 infection. *N Engl J Med.* 2015;373(27):2599–2607.

58. Berenguer M, Prieto M, Palau A, et al. Severe recurrent hepatitis C after liver retransplantation for hepatitis C virus–related graft cirrhosis. *Liver Transplant.* 2003;9(3):228–235.

59. McCashland T, Watt K, Lyden E, et al. Retransplantation for hepatitis C: results of a US multicenter retransplant study. *Liver Transplant.* 2007;13(9):1246–1253.

60. Fontana RJ, Hughes EA, Appelman H, et al. Case report of successful peginterferon, ribavirin, and daclatasvir therapy for recurrent cholestatic hepatitis C after liver retransplantation. *Liver Transplant.* 2012;18(9):1053–1059.

61. Davies SE, Portmann BC, Aldis PM, et al. Hepatic histological findings after transplantation for chronic hepatitis B virus infection, including a unique pattern of fibrosing cholestatic hepatitis. *Hepatology.* 1991;13(1):150–157.

62. Honda M, Kaneko S, Matsushita E, et al. Cell cycle regulation of hepatitis C virus internal ribosomal entry site–directed translation. *Gastroenterology.* 2000;118(1):152–162.
63. Verna EC, Abdelmessih R, Salomao MA, et al. Cholestatic hepatitis C following liver transplantation: an outcome-based histological definition, clinical predictors, and prognosis. *Liver Transplant.* 2013;19(1):78–88.
64. Pungpapong S, Aqel B, Leise M, et al. Multicenter experience using simeprevir and sofosbuvir with or without ribavirin to treat hepatitis C genotype 1 after liver transplant. *Hepatology.* 2015;61(6):1880–1886.
65. Leroy V, Dumortier J, Coilly A, et al. Efficacy of sofosbuvir and daclatasvir in patients with fibrosing cholestatic hepatitis C after liver transplantation. *Clin Gastroenterol Hepatol.* 2015;13(11):1993–2001. e1992.

Chapter 13

Management of Hepatitis C After a Cure

Daniel Berger and Sheila Eswaran

Benefits of a Sustained Virologic Response

The ultimate goal of hepatitis C virus (HCV) treatment with direct-acting antiviral (DAA) therapy is eradication of the virus and avoidance of complications associated with chronic hepatitis C disease. Achieving sustained virologic response (SVR), defined as an undetectable HCV RNA 12 weeks after the end of treatment, has been shown to provide numerous short- and long-term benefits to patients.[1] Of patients who achieved a SVR, more than 99% have remained free of HCV infection after 5 years.[2] Thus, achieving SVR is considered to be a virologic cure of HCV infection.

Reduced Liver-Related Morbidity and Mortality

Patients achieving SVR in response to DAA therapy have been shown to have a lower risk of liver-related morbidity and overall mortality when compared to treatment nonresponders. A large meta-analysis showed that patients with SVR are significantly less likely to develop liver-related mortality, such as death as a result of complications of decompensated cirrhosis, hepatocellular carcinoma (HCC), and/or liver transplant when compared to patients who experienced treatment failure.[3] When compared to patients treated without SVR, those who achieved SVR had a decreased incidence of HCC and hepatic decompensation as well as a lower risk of cardiovascular events and bacterial infections.[4] Multiple studies have also shown a reduction in overall mortality compared with HCV-infected patients who have not been treated. When comparing HCV treated patients to the general population, patients cured of HCV had a higher overall mortality rate than the general population; however, most of the increased mortality in the SVR group was related to drug-related causes and death from liver cancer.[5]

Regression of Fibrosis

In regards to immediate effects of treatment, SVR has been shown to halt progression of liver damage. Several studies have shown that SVR induces regression of fibrosis based on biopsy and noninvasive tests of fibrosis, such as transient elastography.[3,6–9] Chan et al. found that treatment of chronic HCV with DAAs was associated with a significant reduction in liver fibrosis, with nearly 50% of patients attaining a 30% improvement in their Fibroscan score at 12 months posttreatment.[10] Improvement in liver stiffness was thought to be due to reduced necroinflammation as well as a regression of fibrosis beyond the initial decrease that was attributed to inflammation associated with viral clearance.

Because of this halt in progression, patients without advanced liver fibrosis (i.e., Metavir stage F0–F2) who achieve SVR should receive standard medical care that is recommended for patients who are not infected with HCV. Despite potential regression of fibrosis, individuals with advanced liver fibrosis (i.e., Metavir stage F3–F4) remain at risk for complications of cirrhosis and require long-term monitoring.

Monitoring Patients with Cirrhosis

Complications of Cirrhosis

Although the rate of morbidity and mortality improves after SVR, patients who have underlying cirrhosis must still be carefully monitored for complications associated with cirrhosis (Table 13.1). This includes screening for esophageal varices and HCC, as well as close monitoring and early diagnosis of hepatic encephalopathy (HE) and ascites.[11]

Because variceal bleeding is a grave complication of cirrhosis that is associated with a very high 1-year mortality rate (57%), all cirrhotic patients should be screened for clinically significant portal hypertension with either endoscopy or noninvasive testing. Patients with a liver stiffness of less than 20 kPa and a platelet count of greater than 150,000/mm^3 have a very low probability (<5%) of having high-risk varices, and esophagogastroduodenoscopy (EGD) can be circumvented.[12] Management of patients with varices is based on presence of clinical decompensation, size of varices, and whether there are high-risk stigmata on endoscopy.[13]

HE is a complex neuropsychiatric abnormality seen in up to 70% of patients with cirrhosis.[14] Patients should be assessed at each visit for clinical signs of overt HE, including sleep–wake cycle reversal, asterixis, memory difficulty, behavior changes, and somnolence. All patients exhibiting signs of HE should be started on therapy to improve cognitive function and health-related quality of life and to lower risk of progression.[15]

Table 13.1 Sustained virologic response (SVR) achieved	
Noncirrhotic (F0–F2 Fibrosis)	Cirrhotic (F3–F4 Fibrosis)
Monitoring for HBV reactivation in coinfected patients	Monitoring for HBV reactivation in coinfected patients
Consider annual HCV RNA testing in high-risk groups (PWID, MSM)	Consider annual HCV RNA testing in high-risk groups (PWID, MSM)
Age-appropriate standard medical care	HCC surveillance every 6 months with abdominal US
	Esophageal varices surveillance

HBV, hepatitis B virus; *HCV*, hepatitis C virus; *MSM*, men who have sex with me; *PWID*, people who inject drugs.

Ascites is the most common complication of cirrhosis. A diagnostic paracentesis should be performed in all patients with recent-onset ascites to assess the serum-ascites albumin gradient (SAAG) to confirm the etiology of ascites as well as to evaluate for spontaneous bacterial peritonitis, defined as a positive ascitic fluid bacterial culture or an ascitic fluid with polymorphonuclear (PMN) leukocyte count of 250 cells/mm^3 or greater. The initial management of ascites includes sodium restriction and diuretics.

Hepatocellular Carcinoma

HCC is a serious complication of HCV infection, particularly in the cirrhotic population. The risk of HCC for patients with advanced fibrosis prior to HCV treatment and who have regression to minimal fibrosis after treatment is not known. In the absence of data, such patients remain at some risk for HCC and should be monitored at regular intervals for the disease. An abdominal ultrasound at 6-month intervals is the current recommendation for HCC surveillance in patients with cirrhosis.

Data from the interferon era concluded that the incidence of HCC in patients with cirrhosis post-SVR was lower than for those with cirrhosis who were persistently viremic.[3,6-9] Results of current post-DAA SVR data are mixed. Two studies published suggested that SVR after DAA therapy did not reduce the occurrence of de novo HCC or recurrence of HCC.[16,17] These findings were met with some criticism due to a short follow-up period and small patient sample size. Subsequently, data from a larger patient cohort and longer follow-up period showed that there was a significant decrease in incidence of HCC in patients achieving SVR (1.93%) compared to those without SVR (8.38%) and that higher rates of HCC are associated with persistent viremia and more advanced portal hypertension, not necessarily the DAA treatment itself.[18] Some reports hypothesize that the rapid HCV suppression by DAA treatment boosts microscopic tumor foci and may lead to more aggressive/infiltrative tumor when it does occur post SVR.

Concomitant Liver Diseases

Hepatitis B Reactivation

Hepatitis B reactivation, defined as an abrupt increase in hepatitis B virus (HBV) replication in a patient with inactive or resolved HBV, is usually triggered by immunosuppressive therapy or immunodeficiency diseases such as HIV. DAA therapy, unlike prior HCV therapy with interferon, does not cause immunosuppression but rather works by inhibiting viral proteins required for HCV replication. Despite this, there have been some concerns about HBV reactivation with DAA therapy.

In October 2016, the U.S. Food and Drug Administration (FDA) released a black box warning about the risk of hepatitis B reactivation with certain DAA agents. Upon reviewing of spontaneous postmarketing cases of HBV reactivation, 29 cases of HBV reactivation were identified within a 20-month period from 2013 to 2016 in patients treated with DAA agents. All cases were temporally related to DAA initiation. Of these cases, two patients died and one required a liver transplant. The mean time from DAA initiation to HBV reactivation was 53 days.[19] Another study showed that HBV-HCV coinfected patients who were positive for HBsAg were more likely to develop hepatitis due to HBV reactivation as opposed to those with occult HBV infection (defined as presence of HBV DNA in the absence of HBsAg) after DAA treatment.[20]

The etiology for HBV reactivation in the setting of HCV treatment is thought to be due to the role of the HCV virus in suppressing HBV reactivation. Studies have shown that HCV superinfection in the setting of chronic HBV can result in HBeAg seroconversion and sometimes clearance of HBsAg. Therefore, clearance of the HCV infection could theoretically ameliorate immune control of HBV replication and result in HBV reactivation.

The benefits of HCV cure with DAA therapy continues to outweigh the risk of HBV reactivation in coinfected patients. However, all patients should be screened for evidence of current or prior HBV infection before initiating treatment with DAAs by measuring HBsAg and anti-HBc. In patients with serologic evidence of HBV infection, baseline HBV DNA should be measured prior to initiation of DAA treatment. Patients who show evidence of current or prior HBV infection should be monitored for clinical and laboratory signs (i.e., HBsAg, HBV DNA, serum aminotransferase levels, bilirubin) of hepatitis flare or HBV reactivation during DAA treatment and posttreatment follow-up. Further studies are needed to determine monitoring frequency, duration of monitoring after SVR, and other risk factors for HBV reactivation.

Other Concomitant Liver Diseases

After SVR, patients who develops persistently elevated liver tests should undergo evaluation for possible other causes of liver disease, such as alcohol use, iron overload, or fatty liver disease. The rate of concomitant liver diseases in patients with hepatitis C is high. For example, steatosis occurs in 30–70% of patients with chronic HCV (Patel 2012),[21] and the prevalence of HCV in patients with alcohol-related liver disease is 15–40%.[22,23] Therefore, it is recommended that such patients be educated about the risk of liver disease and monitored for liver disease progression with periodic clinical evaluation, including physical examinations and blood tests, if indicated. Progression of fibrosis should also be monitored if there appears to be ongoing hepatic injury.

HCV Reinfection

Following successful treatment of hepatitis C with DAA therapy, patients and providers must maintain careful attention toward preventing potential reinfection. As no HCV vaccine currently exists, patients cured of chronic HCV are at risk for reinfection if ever reexposed. Given this fact, it is important for clinicians to remain vigilant in monitoring certain specific patients who may be at higher risk of reinfection than others. Two patient groups have been identified as being at higher risk: people who inject drugs (PWID) and HIV-infected men who have sex with men.[24] Hill et al. reported a 5-year risk of HCV reinfection of 10.6% in PWID and more than 15% in MSM.[25] In these groups, high-risk behaviors such as illicit drug use and unprotected sexual activity likely lead to increased HCV infection and reinfection rates. Therefore, in addition to HCV treatment, specific focus should be dedicated to behavioral intervention and counseling in an effort to reduce rates of HCV reinfection.

When it comes to monitoring patients who have achieved SVR, those who continue to engage in high-risk behavior should receive at least annual HCV RNA testing to monitor for reinfection, with some studies recommending HIV-positive MSM with prior HCV infection to be tested every 3–5 months for reinfection.[26] After SVR, elevated liver enzymes should trigger a prompt evaluation with an HCV RNA test to assess for the diagnosis of an acute HCV reinfection and treatment in high-risk groups as these patients are also most likely to transmit HCV to other persons.

References

1. AASLD-IDSA. Recommendations for testing, managing, and treating hepatitis C. http://www.hcvguidelines.org.
2. Manns MP, Pockros PJ, Norkrans G, et al. Long-term clearance of hepatitis C virus following interferon alpha-2b or peginterferon alpha-2b, alone or in combination with ribavirin. *J Viral Hepat*. 2013;20(8):524–529.
3. Singal A, Volk M, Jensen D. A sustained viral response is associated with reduced liver-related morbidity and mortality in patients with hepatitis C virus. *Clin Gastroenterol Hepatol*. 2010.8;3:280–288
4. Nahon P, Bourcier V, Layese R, et al. Eradication of hepatitis C virus infection in patients with cirrhosis reduces risk of liver and non-liver complications. *Gastroenterology*. 2017.152;1:142–156.
5. Innes H, McDonald S, Hayes P, et al. Mortality in hepatitis C patients who achieve a sustained viral response compared to the general population. *J Hepatol*. 2017.66;1:19–27
6. Morisco F, Granata R, Stroffolini T, et al. Sustained virological response: a milestone in the treatment of chronic hepatitis C. *World J Gastroenterol*. 2013 May 14;9(18):2793–2798.
7. Morgan TR, Ghany MG, Kim HY, et al. Outcome of sustained virological responders with histologically advanced chronic hepatitis C. *Hepatology*. 2010;52(3):833–844.
8. George SL, Bacon BR, Brunt EM, et al. Clinical, virologic, histologic, and biochemical outcomes after successful HCV therapy: a 5-year follow-up of 150 patients. *Hepatology*. 2009;49(3):729–738.
9. Morgan RL, Baack B, Smith BD, et al. Eradication of hepatitis C virus infection and the development of hepatocellular carcinoma: a meta-analysis of observational studies. *Ann Intern Med*. 2013;158(5 Pt 1):329–337.
10. Chan J, Gogela N, Zheng H. Direct acting anti-viral therapy for chronic hepatitis C virus infection is associated with regression of liver fibrosis, assessed by serial transient elastography (fibroscan). IDWeek abstract 2016.
11. Grewal P, Martin P. Care of the cirrhotic patient. *Clin Liver Dis*. 2009.13; 2:330–340.
12. Garcia-Tsao G, Abraldes JG, Berzigotti A, Bosch J. Portal hypertensive bleeding in cirrhosis: risk stratification, diagnosis, and management: 2016

practice guidance by the American Association for the study of liver diseases. *Hepatology*. 2017 Jan;65(1):310–335.

13. Merli M, Nicolini G, Angeloni S, et al. Incidence and natural history of small esophageal varices in cirrhotic patients. *J Hepatology.* 2003.38;3:266–272

14. Riordan S, Williams R. Treatment of hepatic encephalopathy. *N Engl J Med.* 1997.337;7:473–479.

15. Prasad S, Dhiman R, Duseja A. Lactulose improves cognitive functions and health-related quality of life in patients with cirrhosis who have minimal hepatic encephalopathy. *Hepatology*. 2007.45;3:549–559

16. Conti F, Buonfiglioli F, Scuteri A, et al. Early occurrence and recurrence of hepatocellular carcinoma in HCV-related cirrhosis treated with direct-acting antivirals. *J Hepatol*. 2016.65;4:727–733.

17. Reig M, Marino Z, Perello C, et al. Unexpected high rate of early tumor recurrence in patients with HCV-related HCC undergoing interferon-free therapy. *J Hepatol*. 2016.65;4:719–726.

18. Romano A, Capra F, Piovesan S, et al. Incidence and pattern of "de novo" hepatocellular carcinoma in HCV patients treated with oral DAAs. AASLD abstract 2016.

19. Bersoff-Matcha S, Cao K, Jason M, et al. Hepatitis B reactivation associated with direct acting antiviral therapy for hepatitis C: a review of spontaneous post-marketing cases. AASLD 2016 abstract.

20. Wang C, Ji D, Chen J, et al. Hepatitis due to reactivation of hepatitis B virus in endemic areas among patients with hepatitis C treated with direct-acting antiviral agents. *Clin Gastroenterol Hepatol*. 2017.15;1:132–136.

21. Patel A, Harrison SA. Hepatitis C virus infection and nonalcoholic steatohepatitis. *Gastroenterol Hepatol*. 2012 May;8(5):305–312.

22. Nalpas B, Thiers V, Pol S, et al. Hepatitis C viremia and anti-HCV antibodies in alcoholics. *J Hepatol*. 1992;14:381.

23. Butt AA, Justice AC, Skanderson M, et al. Rate and predictors of treatment prescription for hepatitis C. *Gut*. 2007;56:385.

24. Falade-Nwulia O, Sulkowski M. The HCV care continuum does not end with cure: a call to arms for the prevention of reinfection. *J Hepatol*. 2017.66;2:267–269.

25. Simmons B, Saleem J, Hill A, et al. Risk of late relapse or reinfection with hepatitis C virus after achieving a sustained virological response: a systematic review and meta-analysis. *Clin Infect Dis*. 2016.62;6:683–694.

26. Ingiliz P, Martin T, Rodger A, et al. HCV reinfection incidence and spontaneous clearance rates in HIV-positive men who have sex with men in Western Europe. *J Hepatol*. 2017.66;2:282–287.

Chapter 14

Lexicon of Trials

Deeksha Seth, Sujit V. Janardhan, and Archita P. Desai

Currently Approved Therapies

In this section, we present outline summaries of select phase III trials of currently approved treatment regimens for chronic hepatitis C. Treatment regimens are presented in order of approval by the US Food and Drug Administration (FDA).

Sofosbuvir (NS5B Inhibitor)

NEUTRINO and FISSION Trials (Copublished)
Lawitz E, Mangia A, Wyles D, et al. Sofosbuvir for previously untreated chronic hepatitis C infection. *N Engl J Med.* 2013 May 16;368(20):1878–1887.

NEUTRINO
Study description: Open-label, single-arm, phase III
Patient population: TN, HCV GT1, GT4, GT5, or GT6 (*n* = 327)
Study arms: 12-week course of SOF plus PEG-IFN plus weight-based RBV
Results/ SVR12:
Overall: 90%; all subgroups 80% or greater
Cirrhosis: 80%; GT1b: 82%
Viral resistance to SOF was not detected
Significance: Established the high efficacy of sofosbuvir when added to PEG-IFN in GT1 patients

FISSION
Study description: Randomized, open-label, active-control, phase III
Patient population: TN, GT2 or GT3 (1:3), ~20% with cirrhosis (*n* = 499)
Study arms: 1:1 randomization of 12 weeks of SOF plus RBV (Arm 1) or 24 weeks of PEG-IFN plus RBV (Arm 2)
Results/SVR:
Overall: 67% in Arms 1 and 2
GT2: Arm 1: 97%; Arm 2: 78%
GT3: Arm 1: 56%; Arm 2: 63%

Abbreviations used: *CKD*, chronic kidney disease; *DAA*, direct-acting antivirals; *DCV*, daclatasvir; *EBR*, elbasvir; *ESRD*, end-stage renal disease; *GLE*, glecaprevir; *GT*, genotype; *GZR*, grazoprevir; *HAART*, highly active antiretroviral therapy; *HCC*, hepatocellular carcinoma; *HCV*, hepatitis C virus; *IFN*, interferon; *LED*, lediapsvir; *OAT*, opioid agonist therapy; *OBV*, ombitasvir; *PEG-IFN*, pegylated interferon; *PIB*, pibrentasvir; *PTV*, paritaprevir; *r*, ritonavir; *RAS*, resistance-associated substitutions; *RBV*, ribavirin; *SIM*, simeprevir; *SOF*, sofosbuvir; *SVR*, sustained virologic response; *TE*, treatment-experienced; *TN*, treatment-naïve; *VEL*, velpatasvir; *VOX*, voxilaprevir.

Cirrhosis: Arm 1: 47%; Arm 2: 38%

Significance: Established the efficacy of 12-week regimen of SOF plus RBV for TN GT2 HCV infected patients over PEG-IFN plus RBV. Both the regimens showed poor efficacy in GT3 HCV and cirrhotic patients.

FUSION and POSITRON Trials (Copublished)

Jacobson IM, Gordon SC, Kowdley KV, et al, Sofosbuvir for hepatitis C genotype 2 or 3 in patients without treatment options. *N Engl J Med*. 2013 May 16;368(20):1867–77.

FUSION

Study description: Multicenter, double-blinded, active-controlled, phase III
Patient population: GT2 or GT3, nonresponse to previous IFN-containing regimen, 34% cirrhosis ($n = 201$)
Study arms: 1:1 randomization to SOF and weight-based RBV for 16 weeks ($n = 98$) or for 12 weeks ($n = 103$) followed by 4 weeks of placebo
Results/SVR12:

Overall: 12 weeks: 50%; 16 weeks: 73%; cirrhosis: 12 weeks: 31%; 16 weeks: 66%

GT2: 12 weeks: 86%; 16 weeks: 94%; with cirrhosis: 12 weeks: 60%; 16 weeks: 78%

GT3: 12 weeks: 30%; 16 weeks: 62%; with cirrhosis: 12 weeks: 19%; 16 weeks: 61%

Well-tolerated with similar serious adverse event rates between 12 (5%) and 16 (3%) weeks

Significance: Established the efficacy of a 12-week course of SOF plus RBV in noncirrhotic patients with GT2 HCV as well as the poor performance of this regimen in patients with cirrhosis or GT3 infection in whom extension to 16 weeks marginally improved SVR12 rates

POSITRON

Study description: Randomized, double-blind, placebo-controlled, phase III
Patient population: GT2 or GT3, unable to receive PEG-IFN–based therapy due to unwillingness, intolerance, or medical contraindication, mostly TN (82%), 16% cirrhosis ($n = 278$)
Study arms: 3:1 Randomization to 12 weeks of either SOF plus weight-based RBV ($n = 207$) or placebo ($n = 71$)
Results/SVR12:

78% with SOF plus RBV arm

93% with GT2 compared to 61% with GT3

Significance: Established the efficacy of a 12-week course of SOF plus RBV in patients with GT2 infection and highlighted low efficacy in GT3 infection.

VALENCE Trial

Zeuzem S, Dusheiko GM, Salupere R, et al. Sofosbuvir and Ribavirin in HCV Genotypes 2 and 3. *N Engl J Med*. 2014;370:1993–2001.

Study description: Descriptive, placebo controlled, phase III
Patient population: TE (58%) or TN, GT2 and GT3, 21% with cirrhosis ($n = 419$)

Study arms: SOF plus RBV for 12 weeks in GT2 patients or 24 weeks in GT3 patients
Results/SVR12:
GT2: 93% with 12 weeks SOF plus RBV
78% in TE cirrhotic patients; 94–100% in either TN or TE without cirrhosis
GT3: 85% with 24 weeks SOF plus RBV
TN: 92% with cirrhosis, 95% without cirrhosis
TE: 62% with cirrhosis, 87% without cirrhosis
Significance: Established the efficacy of the regimen of SOF plus RBV for 12 weeks in TN or TE GT2 HCV patients; whereas in hard-to-treat cirrhotic GT3 TE patients, a low but improved SVR12 was observed when extended to 24 weeks of therapy.

SOFOSBUVIR + LEDIPASVIR
(NS5B Inhibitor + NS5A Inhibitor)

ION-2 Trial
Afdhal N, Reddy R, Nelson DR, et al. Ledipasvir and sofosbuvir for previously treated HCV genotype 1 infection. *N Engl J Med*. 2014;370:1483–1493.

Study description: Randomized, open-label, phase III
Patient population: TE (IFN-based ± protease inhibitor), GT1 HCV-infected patients, up to 20% cirrhotic ($n = 440$)
Study arms: Randomized (1:1:1:1) to 12 or 24 weeks of LED and SOF with or without weight-based RBV
Results/SVR12:
Overall: 12 weeks: 94–96%; 24 weeks: 99%
Similar SVR12 among GT1a, GT1b, TE, nonresponders, or prior relapse
Cirrhotic patients: 82–86% with 12 weeks; 100% with 24 weeks
Virologic relapse: 2% after 12 weeks of therapy, none after 24 weeks
3–6% serious adverse events noted in 24 week regimen, none in 12 week.
Significance: The regimen for 12 weeks of LED/SOF in treating noncirrhotic TE patients with GT1 HCV was effective, with cirrhotic patients benefiting with extension of therapy to 24 weeks with no additional benefits of adding RBV.

ION Trial
Afdhal N, Seuzem S, Kwo P, et al. Ledipasvir and sofosbuvir for untreated HCV genotype 1 infection. *N Engl J Med*. 2014;370:1889–1898.

Study description: Randomized, open-label, phase III
Patient population: TN GT1 patients, up to 20% cirrhotic ($n = 870$)
Study arms: Randomized (1:1:1:1) to 12 or 24 weeks of LED/SOF once daily with or without weight-based RBV
Results/SVR12:
Overall: >95% in all arms
Cirrhosis: 94–100%
No effect of baseline nonstructural protein 5A resistance-associated variants (NS5A RAVs)
Virologic failure: <1% of the total patients

Serious adverse events noted: 4% overall (3% in the 24 week arms); discontinuation: 1% in the 24-week arms
Significance: Established 12 weeks of LED/SOF as a highly effective therapy in TN patients with HCV GT1 infection, including those with cirrhosis, with no additional benefit observed on addition of RBV or extending the therapy to 24 weeks even in patients with cirrhosis.

ION-3 Trial

Kowdley K, Gordon SC, Reddy R, et al. Ledipasvir and sofosbuvir for 8 or 12 weeks for chronic HCV without cirrhosis. *N Engl J Med*. 2014;370:1879–1888.

Study description: Randomized, multicenter, open-label, phase III
Patient population: TN noncirrhotic, GT1 HCV-infected patients ($n = 647$)
Study arms: Randomized (1:1:1). LED/SOF for 8 weeks with or without weight-based RBV, or LED and SOF alone for 12 weeks
Results/SVR12:
Overall for 8 weeks: 93% (with RBV) and 94% (without RBV); 12 weeks: 95%
4–5% virologic relapse in patient receiving 8 weeks of therapy; 1% in 12-week group
Subgroup analysis (post-hoc, not in original publication) revealed improved SVR rates of 97 to 100% in the 8-week treatment group if patients had baseline HCV viral load <6 million IU/mL.
NS5A RAV in 18%; SVR12 90%
Serious adverse events: 2% patients; discontinuation: <1% patients
Significance: The study demonstrated the effectiveness of the regimen of LED/SOF in TN GT1 HCV (viral load <6 million IU/mL) infected patients for as short as 8 weeks of therapy with no additional benefit on addition of RBV.

SIMEPREVIR + SOFOSBUVIR (NS3/4A Protease Inhibitor + NS5B Inhibitor)

OPTIMIST-1 Trial

Kwo P, Gitlin N, Nahass R, et al. Simeprevir plus sofosbuvir (12 and 8 weeks) in hepatitis C virus GT1-infected patients without cirrhosis: OPTIMIST-1, a phase III, randomized study. *Hepatology*. 2016 Aug;64(2):370–380.

Study description: Randomized, multicenter, open-label, phase III
Patient population: HCV GT1a/1b infection without cirrhosis, IFN TN or TE ($n = 310$)
Study arms: 1:1 randomization (stratified based on based on GT1 subtype and Q80K polymorphism [GT1b, GT1a with Q80K, GT1a without Q80K]), prior HCV treatment history, and IL28B genotype [CC, non-CC]) to SIM/SOF for 8 or 12 weeks
Results/SVR12:
97% in 12-week arm; 83% in 8-week arm
No discontinuation due to adverse events
Significance: Established 12 weeks of SIM/SOF as the first all-oral treatment for patients infected with GT1 HCV including those with a Q80K polymorphism (These agents had been individually approved prior to this study being published. Their combined efficacy as the "first" all-oral therapy was noted in the phase 2 COSMOS trial published in 2014.)

OPTIMIST-2 Trial

Lawitz E, Matusow G, DeJesus E, et al. Simeprevir plus SOF in patients with chronic hepatitis C virus genotype 1 infection and cirrhosis: A phase 3 study. *Hepatology*. 2016 Aug;64(2):360–369.

Study description: Multicenter, open-label, single-arm, phase III
Patient population: TN or TE GT1 HCV infected patients with compensated cirrhosis ($n = 103$)
Study arms: 12 weeks of SIM/SOF
Results./SVR12:
Overall: 83%; TN: 88%; TE: 79%
Serious adverse events in 5% with discontinuation in 3%
Significance: A high SVR12 was observed in GT1 cirrhotic patients with the above regimen for 12 weeks but was comparatively lower to the other emerging therapies at the time, especially in TE patients. There was discordance from the COSMOS trial (see Other Interesting Trials section), which showed an efficacy of more than 90% for 12 or 24 weeks in cirrhotic patients with or without RBV.

VIEKIRA PAK (Ombitasvir-Paritaprevir-Ritonavir and Dasabuvir) and TECHNIVIE (Ombitasvir, Paritaprevir and Ritonavir) (NS5A Inhibitor + NS3/4A PI + CY3A4/PI + NS5B Inhibitor)

SAPPHIRE-I Trial

Feld JJ, Kowdley KV, Coakley E, et al. Treatment of HCV with ABT-450/r-ombitasvir and dasabuvir with ribavirin. *N Engl J Med*. 2014 Apr 24;370(17): 1594–1603.

Study description: Randomized, multicenter, double-blind, placebo-controlled, phase III
Patient population: TN and noncirrhotic HCV GT1 ($n = 631$)
Study arms: 3:1 ratio. Arm 1: Single-tablet coformulation of ABT-450 (paritaprevir or PTV)/ritonavir (r)/ombitasvir (OBV) and dasabuvir with RBV; and Arm 2: Matching placebo regimen for 12 weeks
Results/SVR12:
Overall 96.2%
95.3% (GT1a); 98% (GT1b)
0.2% virologic failure; 1.5% relapse after treatment
Rate of discontinuation in each arm: 0.6%.
Significance: A multitargeted regimen of OBV/PTV/r and dasabuvir with RBV for 12 weeks was highly effective in TN noncirrhotic patients with HCV GT1 infection.

SAPPHIRE-II Trial

Zeuzam S, Jacobson IM, Baykal T, et al. Retreatment of HCV with ABT-450/r-ombitasvir and dasabuvir with ribavirin. *N Engl J Med*. 2014 Apr 24; 370(17):1604–1614.

Study description: Randomized, multicenter, double-blind, phase III
Patient population: TE noncirrhotic HCV GT1 (PEG-IFN-RBV with relapse, a partial response, or a null response; $n = 394$)

Study arms: 3:1 ratio coformulated OBV/PTV/r and dasabuvir with RBV or matching placebos for 12 weeks
Results/SVR12:
Overall: 96.3%
Prior relapse: 95.3%; partial response: 100%; and prior null response: 95.2%
Serious adverse events: 2%; 1% with placebo
Discontinuation: 1%
Significance: Established the efficacy of the above regimen for 12 weeks among TE noncirrhotic HCV GT1-infected patients, including those with a prior null response.

TURQUOISE-II Trial

Poordad F, Hezode C, Trinh R, et al. ABT-450/r-ombitasvir and dasabuvir with ribavirin for hepatitis C with cirrhosis. *N Engl J Med.* 2014 May 22;370(21):1973–1982.

Study description: Randomized, multicenter, open-label, controlled, phase III study
Patient population: TN or TE (PEG-IFN and RBV) patients with chronic HCV GT1 infection and Child Turcotte Pugh (CTP) A cirrhosis ($n = 380$)
Study arms: Treatment with OBV/PTV/r, dasabuvir and weight-based RBV for 12 weeks (Arm 1) and 24 weeks (Arm 1)
Results/SVR12:
91.8% in Arm 1; 95.9% in Arm 2
HCV GT1a: 89% in Arm 1; 94% in Arm 2
HCV GT1b: 99% in Arm 1; 100% in Arm 2
Overall serious adverse events: 5.5%; discontinuation: 2.1%
Significance: Established the efficacy of OBV/PTV/r, dasabuvir with RBV for 24 weeks rather than 12 weeks in TN or TE HCV GT1 patients.

PEARL-III AND PEARL-IV TRIALS (Co-published)

Ferenci P, Bernstein D, Lalezani J, et al. ABT-450/r-ombitasvir and dasabuvir with or without RBV for HCV. *N Engl J Med.* 2014;370:1983–1992.

Study description: Randomized, double-blind, placebo-controlled, phase III
Patient population: TN PEARL-III: HCV GT1b ($n = 419$); PEARL IV: HCV GT1a ($n = 305$)
Study arms: Randomized into two arms: OBV/PTV/r and dasabuvir with (Arm 1) or without (Arm 2) RBV for 12 weeks.
Results/SVR12:
PEARL-III: 99.5% in Arm 1; 99% in Arm 2 with 1 virologic failure
Serious adverse events: 1% in each arm
PEARL-IV: 97% in Arm 1; 90.2% in Arm 2 with virologic failure of 7.8% without RBV and 2% with RBV
Discontinuation due to adverse events: <1%
Serious adverse events: 1%
Significance: Established the efficacy of the above regimen for 12 weeks in TN HCV GT1 patients with less virologic failures noted in the GT1a patients on addition of RBV to the regimen.

PEARL-II Trial

Andreone P, Colombo MG, Enejosa JV, et al. ABT-450, ritonavir, ombitasvir, and dasabuvir achieve 97% and 100% sustained virologic response with or without ribavirin in treatment-experienced patients with HCV GT1b infection. *Gastroenterology.* 2014 Aug;147(2):359–365.

Study description: Randomized, multicenter, open-label, phase III
Patient population: HCV GT1b, noncirrhotic, TE PEG-IFN and RBV ($n = 179$)
Study arms: 1:1 randomization. OBV/PTV/r and dasabuvir with (Arm 1) and without (Arm 2) RBV for 12 weeks.
Results/SVR12:
Arm 1: 96.6%; Arm 2: 100%
No virologic failures noted.
Significance: Established a high rate of SVR12 with this IFN-free regimen in TE HCV GT1b-infected patients.

TURQUOISE-III Trial

Feld JJ, Moreno C, Trinh R, et al. Sustained virologic response of 100% in HCV GT1b patients with cirrhosis receiving ombitasvir/paritaprevir/r and dasabuvir for 12 weeks. *J Hepatol.* 2016 Feb;64(2):301–307.

Study description: Descriptive, multicenter, open-label, phase III
Patient population: TN and TE (PEG-IFN/RBV) HCV GT1b with CTP Class A cirrhosis ($n = 60$)
Study arms: 12 weeks of OBV/PTV/r and dasabuvir
Results/SVR12:
Overall: 100%
TN: 97.9%; TE: 96.2%
Serious adverse events: 1.7%
Significance: The RBV-free regimen of OBV/PTV/r and dasabuvir for 12 weeks was well tolerated among HCV GT1b cirrhotic patients with low rate of adverse events.

AGATE-I Trial

Asselah T, Hezode C, Qaqish RB, et al. Ombitasvir, paritaprevir, and ritonavir plus Ribavirin in adults with hepatitis C virus genotype 4 infection and cirrhosis (AGATE-I): A multicenter, phase III, randomised open-label trial. *Lancet Gastroenterol Hepatol.* 2016 Sep;1(1):25–35.

Study description: Randomized, multicenter, open-label, phase III
Patient population: TE and TN (PEG-IFN and RBV) HCV GT4 infection and compensated cirrhosis ($n = 120$)
Study arms: 1:1 randomization to receive OBV/PTV/r with weight-based RBV for either 12 weeks ($n = 59$) or 16 weeks ($n = 61$), stratified by HCV treatment history and by type of nonresponse to previous HCV treatment
Results/SVR12:
Overall for 12-week: 97%; 16-week: 98%
Virologic breakthrough in 12-week group: 2%
Significance: The above regimen for 12 weeks was found to be effective in HCV GT4 infection and compensated cirrhosis with no additional benefit to extension of therapy to 16 weeks.

GARNET Trial

Welzel TM, Asselah T, Dumas EO, et al. Ombitasvir, paritaprevir, and ritonavir plus dasabuvir for 8 weeks in previously untreated patients with hepatitis C virus genotype 1b infection without cirrhosis (GARNET): A single-arm, open-label, phase 3b trial. *Lancet Gastroenterol Hepatol.* 2017 Jul;2(7):494–500.

Study description: Multicenter, open-label, single-arm, phase IIIb
Patient population: TN noncirrhotic HCV GT1b ($n = 163$)
Study arms: Once-daily OBV/PTV/r with twice-daily dasabuvir for 8 weeks.
Results/SVR12:
SVR12: 98%
F0–F2: 99%; F3: 87%
55% with baseline polymorphism, presence of RAVs did not impact SVR12: >94%
Virologic failure: 1%
Discontinuation due to adverse events: <1%
Significance: Established the efficacy of OBV/PTV/r with dasabuvir therapy for as short as 8 weeks for TN noncirrhotic HCV GT1b-infected patients.

DACLATASVIR (NS5A Inhibitor)

ALLY-3 Trial

Nelson DR, Cooper JN, Lalezari JP, et al. All-oral 12-week treatment with daclatasvir plus Sofosbuvir in patients with hepatitis C virus genotype 3 infection: ALLY-3 phase III study. *Hepatology.* 2015 Apr;61(4):1127–1135.

Study description: Open-label, two-cohort, phase II
Patient population: Chronic HCV GT3 infection, TN ($n = 101$) and TE ($n = 51$), with ($n = 32$) and without ($n = 109$) compensated cirrhosis ($N = 152$)
Study arms: Two cohorts: Both received DCV plus SOF for 12 weeks
Results/SVR12:
TN: 90% (97% without cirrhosis); TE 86% (94% without cirrhosis)
Cirrhosis: 63% vs. no cirrhosis: 96%
Significance: 12-week regimen of DCV/SOF was well-tolerated and effective in noncirrhotic GT3 HCV-infected patients. The therapy was far less effective in patients with cirrhosis.

ALLY-3+ Trial

Leroy V, Angus P, Bronowicki JP, et al. Daclatasvir, sofosbuvir, and ribavirin for hepatitis C virus genotype 3 and advanced liver disease: A randomized phase III study. *Hepatology.* 2016 May;63(5):1430–1441.

Study description: Open-label, randomized trial, phase III
Patient population: Chronic HCV GT3 infection, TN ($n = 13$) and TE ($n = 37$) with advanced fibrosis ($n = 14$) and compensated cirrhosis ($n = 36$; $N = 50$)
Study arms: Randomized 1:1 to DCV, SOF, and weight-based RBV for 12 weeks or 16 weeks
Results/SVR12:
Overall: 90% (88% in 12-week and 92% in 16-week)
Advanced fibrosis: 100%; cirrhosis: 86% (12-week: 83%, 16-week: 89%)
TE with cirrhosis was 87%
8% relapsed; no virological breakthroughs

Significance: Established the efficacy of addition of RBV to a 12-week therapy of DCV/SOF for effective treatment of GT3 HCV-infected patients with cirrhosis.

ALLY-1 Trial

Poordad F, Schiff ER, Vierling JM. Daclatasvir with sofosbuvir and ribavirin for hepatitis C virus infection with advanced cirrhosis or post-liver transplantation recurrence. *Hepatology*. 2016 May;63(5):1493–1505.

Some patients with compensated cirrhosis were included in this trial (20%). Please refer to the section "The Hard to Treat Population: Decompensated Cirrhosis,: for trial details.

ZEPATIER (ELBASVIR and GRAZOPREVIR) (NS5A Inhibitor + NS3/4A PI)

C-EDGE Treatment-Naïve Trial

Zeuzem S, Ghalib R, Reddy KR, et al. Grazoprevir-elbasvir combination therapy for treatment-naive cirrhotic and noncirrhotic patients with chronic hepatitis C virus genotype 1, 4, or 6 infection: A randomized trial. *Ann Intern Med*. 2015 Jul 7;163(1):1–13.

Study description: Randomized, blinded, placebo-controlled, parallel-group, phase III
Patient population: Cirrhotic and noncirrhotic, TN GT1, GT4, or GT6 chronic HCV (N = 421)
Study arms: Randomized 3:1 to immediate or deferred therapy. Fixed-dose grazoprevir (GZR), elbasvir (EBR) for 12 weeks was administered, stratified by fibrosis and GT. After 4 weeks of follow-up, placebo recipients were non-blinded and given EBR/GZR open label
Results/SVR12:
Overall: 95% with immediate treatment
GT1a: 92%; GT1b: 99%; GT4: 100%; GT6: 80%
With cirrhosis: 97%; without cirrhosis: 94%
Baseline HCV RNA Levels: ≤800K IU/mL: 100%; >800K IU/mL: 92%
Baseline NS5A RAVs and SVR12 in GT1:
GT1a: Baseline NS5A RAVs, 58%; no baseline NS5A RAVs, 99%
GT1b: Baseline NS5A RAVs, 94%; no baseline NS5A RAVs, 100%
Virologic failure: 3%, breakthrough infection: <1%
No serious adverse events related to the study drug.
Significance: Established the efficacy of all-oral, fixed combination of grazoprevir-elbasvir regimen in TN cirrhotic and noncirrhotic patients with HCV GT1, GT4, or GT6 infection with viral relapse occurring in 12 patients due to baseline NS5A polymorphisms and emergent nonstructural protein 3 (NS3) or NS5A variants or both.

C-EDGE Treatment-Experienced Trial

Kwo P, Gane EJ, Cheng-Yuan P, et al. Effectiveness of elbasvir and grazoprevir combination, with or without RBV, for treatment-experienced patients with chronic hepatitis C infection. *Gastroenterology*. 2017;152(1):164–175.

Study description: Randomized, open-label, parallel-group, phase III

Patient population: TE (PEG-IFN plus RBV treatment failure), cirrhotic and noncirrhotic, GT1, GT4, or GT6 chronic HCV ($N = 420$)
Study arms: Oral, once-daily, fixed-dose GZR/EBR with or without RBV for 12 or 16 weeks
Results/SVR12:
SVR12 by treatment duration and regimen: 12 weeks: without RBV: 92%; with RBV: 94%; 16-week: without RBV: 92%; with RBV: 98%
SVR12 in GT1a: 95%, GT1b: 98.6%, GT4: 88.9%
GT1a: 12 weeks: 90–93%; 16 weeks 94–95%
With cirrhosis: 89% vs. without cirrhosis: 92–100%
Virologic failure in 7.5% of GT1 and GT4 patients with previous null response to PEG-IFN, 0% with previous relapse
Of the 10/12, GT1a with virologic failure had a baseline NS5A RAV
SVR12 rates were 97.2% in patients without baseline NS3 RAVs and 94.3% with NS3 RAVs.
RAVs did not seem to impact SVR12 among patients with HCV GT1b, GT4, or GT6 infection
Significance: Established the efficacy of the regimen of grazoprevir/elbasvir with or without RBV for 12 or 16 weeks in patients with HCV GT1, GT4, or GT6 infections with previous failure to PEG-IFN plus RBV therapy.

SOFOSBUVIR + VELPATASVIR
(NS5B Inhibitor + NS5A Inhibitor)

ASTRAL-1 Trial
Feld JJ, Jacobson IM, Hezode C, et al. Sofosbuvir and velpatasvir for HCV genotype 1, 2, 4, 5, and 6 infection. *N Engl J Med.* 2015 Dec 31;373(27):2599–2607.

Study description: Randomized, multicenter, double-blind, placebo-controlled, phase III
Patient population: TN and TE (excluding those previously treated with NS5A or NS5B inhibitor), GT1, GT2, GT4, GT5, or GT6 with or without compensated cirrhosis ($n = 624$)
Study arms: SOF-VEL or placebo in 5:1 ratio for 12 weeks.
Results/SVR12:
Overall: 99% with a range of 97–100% across the genotypes with 2 viral relapses in patients with GT1a and 1b.
Cirrhotic and TE: >99%
No effect of baseline NS5A resistance-associated variants (42%)
Significance: Established the efficacy of a 12-week course of SOF/VEL in patients with non-GT3 HCV infection, including patients who were TE and for those with compensated cirrhosis.

ASTRAL-2 and ASTRAL-3 Trials (Co-published)
Foster GR, Afdhal N, Stuart K, et al. Sofosbuvir and velpatasvir for HCV genotype 2 and 3 infection. *N Engl J Med.* 2015;373:2608–2617.

ASTRAL-2 Trial

Study description: Randomized, multicenter, open-label, phase III
Patient population: TE and TN GT2, including patients with compensated cirrhosis (14%) ($n = 266$)

Study arms: Randomized into two arms according to presence or absence of cirrhosis and previous treatment: SOF/VEL or SOF plus RBV for 12 weeks
Results/SVR12:
99% for SOF/VEL versus 94% with SOF-RBV
SOF/VEL: TE or TN with or without cirrhosis: 99–100%
SOF-RBV: TE noncirrhotic: 81%; 93–100% in rest of the subgroups
Significance: SOF/VEL (without RBV) was more effective than SOF-RBV among the TE and TN HCV GT2 patients, including those with compensated cirrhosis.

ASTRAL-3 Trial
Study description: Randomized, open-label, phase III
Patient population: TE or TN GT3 with or without compensated cirrhosis ($n = 552$)
Study arms: SOF/VEL for 12 weeks vs. SOF plus RBV for 24 weeks
Results/SVR12:
Overall 95% with SOF/VEL vs. 80% with SOF plus RBV
Cirrhotic: TE 89%; TN 93%
Baseline NS5A resistance associated variants 88% versus 97% without baseline resistance
Significance: Established the efficacy of a 12-week regimen of SOF/VEL in patients with chronic HCV GT3 infection over SOF-RBV for 24 weeks. Demonstrated lower SVR in TE cirrhotic patients and those with baseline NS5A RAVs.

Agents Under Investigation

In this section, we present capsule summaries of available data regarding direct-acting antivirals (DAAs) that are not yet approved by the US Food and Drug Administration (FDA) for the treatment of chronic hepatitis C but carry great promise and are likely to be of clinical importance in the coming years. For many of these agents, trials are ongoing, and data are only available in abstract form.

UPRIFOSBUVIR + GRAZOPREVIR + RUZASVIR (NS5B Inhibitor + NS3/4A PI + NS5A Inhibitor)

C-Crest Trials 1 and 2 Parts A–C

Gane EJ, Pianko S, Robert SK, et al. Safety and efficacy of an 8-week regimen of grazoprevir plus ruzasvir plus uprifosbuvir compared with grazoprevir plus elbasvir plus uprifosbuvir in participants without cirrhosis infected with hepatitis C virus genotypes 1, 2, or 3 (C-CREST-1 and C-CREST-2, part A): two randomised, phase 2, open-label trials. *Lancet Gastroenterol Hepatol*. 2017;2(11):805–813.

Gane EJ, Pianko S, Roberts SK, et al. EASL, 2016. High efficacy of an 8-week drug regimen of grazoprevir/MK-8408/MK-3682 in HCV genotype 1, 2 and 3-infected patients. (C-CREST 1 & 2). *J Hepatol*. 2016;64(2):S759.

Lawitz E, Buti M, Vierling JM, et al. Safety and efficacy of a fixed-dose combination regimen of grazoprevir, ruzasvir, and uprifosbuvir with or without ribavirin in participants with and without cirrhosis with chronic hepatitis C virus genotype 1, 2, or 3 infection (C-CREST-1 and C-CREST-2, part B): two randomised, phase 2, open-label trials. *Lancet Gastroenterol Hepatol*. 2017;2(11):814–823.

Wyles D, Wedemeyer H, Ben-Ari Z, et al. Grazoprevir, ruzasvir, and uprifosbuvir for hepatitis C virus after NS5A treatment failure. *Hepatology*. 2017;66(6):1794–1804.

These are randomized, open-label, phase II studies which evaluated the efficacy of the MK-3682B (three-drug coformulation of polymerase inhibitor [MK-3682], protease inhibitor GZR plus NS5A inhibitor ruzasvir [MK-8408] with and without RBV at varying doses for treatment of HCV GT1, GT2, and GT3 [N = 928]). The treatment periods studied were 8, 12, or 16 weeks. GT1, GT2, and GT3 patients were TN noncirrhotic except in part B, which also included 44% of GT3 patients who were TE and had previously failed IFN/RBV, along with 38% of patients with cirrhosis. With 8 weeks of treatment, SVR12 and SVR24 were as follows: GT1: 98–100%; GT2: 94% with MK-3682 450 mg/GZR/MK-8408 and <71% in the other arms; GT3: 86–95%. With the 12-week therapy, SVR12 were as follows: GT1: 99%; GT2: 97%; GT3: 97%. With the 16-week therapy, SVR 12 was 100% for GT2 and 96% for GT3. SVR12 in patients who relapsed with above drug regimens after 8 weeks of therapy and were retreated with MK-3682B with RBV for 16 weeks was GT1 and 3: 100%; GT2: 93%. Efficacy was comparable in patients with and without cirrhosis. Addition of RBV or the presence of cirrhosis did not have any effect on the SVR12 rates. Less than 4% of patients had serious adverse events, mostly in the RBV arm, with 8% discontinuation observed with 16 weeks of therapy. These study results support the promise of MK-3682B as a safe and effective treatment regimen for GT1, GT2, and GT3 HCV patients.

C-SURGE Trial

Wyles D, Wedemeyer H, Ben-Ari Z, et al. Grazoprevir, ruzasvir, and uprifosbuvir for hepatitis C virus after NS5A treatment failure. *Hepatology*. 2017;66(6):1794–1804.

This is an open-label, phase II study designed to evaluate the safety and efficacy of the MK-3682B regimen in both cirrhotic and noncirrhotic GT1 HCV patients with previous DAA failure with LED/SOF or EBR/GZR. MK-3682B with RBV for 16 weeks or without RBV for 24 weeks was administered and interim analysis was done through SVR8. In the interim analysis, SVR8 was 100% in both arms. Also, a 100% SVR4 rate was observed in all patients reaching follow-up week 4, regardless of baseline RAV presence. No serious adverse event or treatment discontinuations were noted. Thus, in GT1 HCV-infected patients with previous relapse after DAA therapy, with or without compensated cirrhosis, MK-3682B with (RBV for 16 weeks or without RBV for 24 weeks) is established as a highly effective regimen.

SOFOSBUVIR + VELPATASVIR + VOXILAPREVIR
(NS5B Inhibitor + NS5A Inhibitor + NS3/4A PI)

POLARIS-1 Trial

Bourlière M, Gordon SC, Flamm SL, et al. Sofosbuvir, velpatasvir, and voxilaprevir for previously treated HCV infection. *NEJM*. 2017;376(22):2134–2146.

POLARIS-1 was a randomized, double-blind, placebo-controlled phase III study that evaluated sofosbuvir/velpatasvir/voxilaprevir (GS-9857) (SOF/VEL/VOX) in HCV GT1–GT6-infected, NS5A inhibitor-experienced patients (most commonly LED/DCV) with or without cirrhosis for 12 weeks ($n = 263$). 96% SVR12 was achieved in the treatment arm. Virologic failure was not seen in noncirrhotic patients but occurred in 5% of those with cirrhosis. Therefore, SOF/VEL/VOX was effective in TE patients with and without cirrhosis and across all HCV GTs.

POLARIS-2 Trial
Jacobson IM, Lawitz E, Gane EJ, et al. Efficacy of 8 weeks of sofosbuvir, velpatasvir, and voxilaprevir in patients with chronic HCV infection: 2 phase 3 randomized trials. *Gastroenterology*. 2017;153(1):113–122.

In this open-label, randomized, active comparator, phase III trial, GT1–GT6 HCV-infected, TN patients with or without compensated cirrhosis were evaluated for 8 weeks of SOF/VEL/VOX regimen ($n = 501$) versus 12 weeks of SOF/VEL ($n = 440$). SVR12 was 95% in the SOF/VEL/VOX arm versus 98% in the SOF/VEL arm. In cirrhotics, SVR12 was 91% in the SOF/VEL/VOX arm versus 99% in SOF/VEL arm. Relapse rates were higher in the SOF/VEL/VOX arm as compared to the SOF/VEL arm (4% vs. 0.6%), particularly in those with GT1a HCV. Thus, POLARIS 2 concluded that a pan-genotypic regimen of SOF/VEL for 12 weeks is superior to a SOF/VEL/VOX regimen for 8 weeks in TN patients with or without cirrhosis

POLARIS-3 Trial
Jacobson IM, Lawitz E, Gane EJ, et al. Efficacy of 8 weeks of sofosbuvir, velpatasvir, and voxilaprevir in patients with chronic HCV infection: 2 phase 3 randomized trials. *Gastroenterology*. 2017;153(1):113–122.

The POLARIS 3 study enrolled TE and TN cirrhotic patients with GT3 HCV infection. It was an open-label, randomized, active comparator, phase III trial comparing 8 weeks of SOF/VEL/VOX ($n = 110$) versus 12 weeks of SOF/VEL ($n = 109$). SVR12 was 96% in both arms. Both regimens were well tolerated, with frequency of adverse events comparable between the regimens. The SVR12 in TN patients receiving SOF/VEL was 99% versus 96% in patients receiving SOF/VEL/VOX, while a higher SVR12 was observed in TE patients receiving SOF/VEL/VOX (97%) versus 91% in SOF/VEL. Frequency of serious adverse events were rare and comparable between both the arms. Thus, preliminary results from POLARIS 3 establish excellent efficacy of 12-week SOF/VEL for TN and 8-week SOF/VEL/VOX for TE GT3 cirrhotic patients.

POLARIS-4 Trial
Bourlière M, Gordon SC, Flamm SL, et al. Sofosbuvir, velpatasvir, and voxilaprevir for previously treated HCV infection. *NEJM*. 2017;376(22):2134–2146.

This randomized, open-label, active comparator, phase III trial evaluated SOF/VEL/VOX ($n = 182$, only GT4–6) versus SOF/VEL ($n = 151$, GT1–6) for 12 weeks in GT1–6 HCV-infected patients with or without cirrhosis and with prior DAA experience, excluding the NS5A inhibitors. SVR12 rates of 97% (SOF/VEL/VOX) versus 90% (SOF/VEL) were observed. In both regimens, cirrhotic patients had lower SVR12 rates (96% arm 1 vs. 86% arm 2) as compared to the noncirrhotic patients (98% arm 1 vs. 94% arm 2). In the SOF/VEL arm, two discontinuations were observed due to adverse events and lack of efficacy versus none receiving SOF/VEL/VOX regimen. In this preliminary report, SOF/VEL/VOX is superior to SOF/VEL although both are highly effective pan-genotypic regimens in patients with prior experience with SOF, SIM, deleobuvir, telaprevir, and mericitabine.

GLECAPREVIR/PIBRENTASVIR
(NS3/4A PI + NS5A Inhibitor)

ENDURANCE Trials 1, 2, 3, and 4

Zeuzem S, Feld J, Wang S, et al, ENDURANCE-1: a phase 3 evaluation of the efficacy and safety of 8- versus 12-week treatment with Glecaprevir/Pibrentasvir (formerly ABT-493/ABT-530) in HCV genotype 1 infected patients with or without HIV-1 co-infection and without cirrhosis. *Hepatology*. 2016;64. [Abstract 253].

Asselah T, Kowdley KV, Zadeikis N, et al. Efficacy of glecaprevir/pibrentasvir for 8 or 12 weeks in patients with Hepatitis C Virus genotype 2, 4, 5, or 6 infection without cirrhosis. *Clin Gastroenterol Hepatol*. 2017 Sep [Epub ahead of print].

Foster GR, Gane E, Asatryan A, et al. Endurance-3: a phase 3, randomized, open-label, active-controlled study to compare efficacy and safety of ABT-493/ABT-530 to sofosbuvir co-administered with daclatasvir in adults with HCV genotype 3 infection. *J Hepatol*. 2016;64:S292.

Glecaprevir (GLE)/pibrentasvir (PIB) is an investigational pan-genotypic regimen currently being evaluated in the ENDURANCE clinical trials, which are multicenter, phase III trials: ENDURANCE-1 (randomized, open-label, 8 [n = 351] and 12 weeks [n = 352], with and without HIV coinfection included), ENDURANCE-2 (randomized, double blind, placebo controlled, 12 weeks, n = 202), ENDURANCE-4 (open-label, single-arm, 12 weeks, n = 121). The ENDURANCE trials evaluated the safety and efficacy of the GLE/PIB regimen in TE or TN noncirrhotic patients with HCV GT1; GT2; and GT4, -5, or -6, respectively. In preliminary reports, more than 99% SVR12 was achieved with almost no virologic failures with the GLE/PIB regimen in the patients in all study arms.

ENDURANCE-3 is an open-label, active-controlled, phase III trial which evaluated the efficacy of GLE/PIB in TN noncirrhotic HCV GT3 patients. The study arms are as follows: Arm 1: 8 weeks with GLE/PIB, nonrandomized, n = 157; Arm 2: 12 weeks with GLE/PIB, randomized, n = 233; Arm 3: 12 weeks with SOF plus DCV, randomized, n = 115. 95% SVR12 was observed with GLE/PIB for 8 or 12 weeks versus 97% with SOF plus DCV for 12 weeks in intention to treat (ITT) population. 3% of patients relapsed in Arm 1 versus 1% in Arms 2 and 3 each. 1% discontinuation observed due to the study drugs in Arms 2 and 3 each. Overall, adverse events were lower at 8 weeks of GLE/PIB than at 12 weeks. The study established the efficacy of the 8-week regimen of GLE/PIB over 12 weeks for TN noncirrhotic HCV GT3 patients.

MAGELLAN-2 Trial

Reau N, Kwo PY, Rhee S. MAGELLAN 2: Safety and efficacy of glecaprevir/pibrentasvir in liver or renal transplant adults with chronic hepatitis C genotype 1-6 infection. EASL International Liver Meeting, April 2017.

MAGELLAN-2 is a multicenter, open-label, single-arm, phase IIIb trial which evaluated the efficacy of the regimen of GLE/PIB for 12 weeks in TN (66%) or TE (34%) (IFN, PEG-IFN, RBV, or SOF) chronic, noncirrhotic, pan-genotypic HCV infection with 3 months post-liver transplantation (80% patients) or post-renal transplantation (20% patients) ($n = 100$). Overall, 98% SVR12 was observed in the ITT group, which was higher than the historical SVR12 of 94%. 2% of the patients had serious adverse events related to the study drug. The study established the efficacy of the regimen of GLE/PIB for 12 weeks in post liver or renal transplant recipients with pan-genotypic HCV infection without cirrhosis irrespective of their treatment status.

SURVEYOR-I and -II Trials

Kwo PY, Poordad F, Asatryan A, et al. Glecaprevir and pibrentasvir yield high response rates in patients with HCV genotype 1–6 without cirrhosis. *J Hepatol*. 2017 Aug;67(2):263–271.

SURVEYOR-I and SURVEYOR-II are open-label, multicenter, phase II trials which evaluated the regimen of GLE/PIB with varying doses with or without RBV for 8 or 12 weeks in TN or TE (PEG-IFN + RBV) noncirrhotic patients with chronic pan-genotypic HCV infection ($n = 449$). SVR12 according to the genotypes with 12 weeks of treatment were: GT1: 97–100%; GT2: 96–100%; GT3: 83–94%; and GT4–6: 100%. With 8 weeks of treatment, SVR12 for GT1, GT2, and GT3 were 97–98%. SURVEYOR-II, parts 2 and 3 also studied the GLE/PIB regimen in HCV GT3 cirrhotic patients and observed an SVR12 rate of >96% for 12 weeks. No serious adverse events occurred due to the study drugs, although <1% patients discontinued treatment due to adverse events. Overall, the 8- or 12-week regimen of GLE/PIB was highly effective and well tolerated in noncirrhotic patients with pan-genotypic HCV infection irrespective of their treatment status, and in GT3, irrespective of the presence of cirrhosis.

The "Hard to Treat" Population

Decompensated Cirrhosis (Pretransplant)

SOLAR-1 Trial

Charlton M, Everson GT, Flamm SL, et al. Ledipasvir and sofosbuvir plus ribavirin for treatment of HCV infection in patients with advanced liver disease. *Gastroenterology*. 2015 Sep;149(3):649–659.

Study description: Randomized, multicenter, open-label, prospective, phase II
Patient population: TN or TE HCV GT1 ($n = 332$) or GT4 ($n = 5$); ($N = 337$)
Study arms: Cohort A = pretransplant patients with cirrhosis and moderate to severe hepatic impairment (CTP Class B or C); Cohort B = post-liver transplantation (CTP Class A, B, or C). Fixed-dose combination of LED/SOF plus RBV for 12 or 24 weeks.
Results/SVR12:
Cohort A: Overall SVR12: 87–89%. CTP B: 87–89%; CTP C: 86–87%
Cohort B: SVR12: No cirrhosis: 96–98%; CTP A: 96%; CTP B: 85–88%; CTP C: 60–75%

Fibrosing cholestatic hepatitis: SVR12 100%

Discontinuations due to adverse events: 4%; deaths: 2.9% mostly from complications related to hepatic decompensation

Significance: LED/SOF plus RBV for 12 weeks produced high rates of SVR12 in patients with advanced liver disease, including those with decompensated cirrhosis before and after liver transplantation.

ASTRAL-4 Trial

Curry MP, O'Leary JG, Bzowej N, et al. Sofosbuvir and velpatasvir for HCV in patients with decompensated cirrhosis. *N Engl J Med*. 2015 Dec 31; 373(27):2618–2628.

Study description: Randomized, open-label, phase III

Patient population: TN or TE GT1, GT2, GT3, GT4, or GT6 with decompensated cirrhosis (CTP class B); ($n = 267$)

Study arms: SOF/VEL for 12 weeks (Arm 1, $n = 90$) or 24 weeks (Arm 2, $n = 90$) or SOF/VEL plus RBV for 12 weeks (Arm 3, $n = 87$)

Results/SVR12:

Arm 1: 88% (GT1), 100% (GT2, 4, 6)

Arm 2: 92% (GT1), 86% (GT2, 4, 6)

Arm 3: 96% (GT1), 100% (GT2, 4, 6)

GT3: Without RBV: 50%; with RBV: 85%

CTP scores improved over baseline in 47%, remain unchanged in 42%, worsened in 11%

Serious adverse events: Arm 1: 19%, Arm 2: 18%; Arm 3: 16%

Discontinuations: Arm 1: 1%, Arm 2: 4%, Arm 3: 4%

Significance: Established the efficacy and safety of a therapeutic regimen of 12 weeks of SOF/VEL in patients with decompensated cirrhosis, with increased efficacy in GT1 patients with the addition of RBV or extension of therapy to 24 weeks and increased efficacy in GT3 patients with the addition of RBV.

ALLY-1 Trial

Poordad F, Schiff ER, Vierling JM, et al. Daclatasvir with sofosbuvir and ribavirin for hepatitis C virus infection with advanced cirrhosis or post-liver transplantation recurrence. *Hepatology*. 2016 May;63(5):1493–1505.

Study description: Multicenter, observational, open-label, phase III

Patient population: TN or TE, GT1 (76%), GT2, GT3, GT4, GT5, GT6 compensated (20%) or decompensated (80%) cirrhosis ($n = 60$) or HCV recurrence posttransplant ($n = 53$; $N = 113$)

Study arms: Two cohorts: Cirrhosis and posttransplant recurrence. Each received DCV/SOF and RBV for 12 weeks with a 24-week follow-up

Results/SVR12:

Cirrhosis: GT1, 82% (1a: 76%, 1b: 100%); GT2, 80%; GT3, 83%; GT4, 100%

CTP A: 93%; B, 94%; C, 56%

CTP score improved in 60%, unchanged in 25%, worsened in 15%

Most prominent improvement in B and C

Posttransplant recurrence: Overall, 94%; GT1, 95%; GT3, 91%

3–4% patients in each cohort discontinued all therapy due to adverse event

Cirrhosis cohort: 17%, posttransplant cohort: 8% discontinuation

No serious adverse events occurred owing to the regimen.

Significance: The pan-genotypic combination of DCV/SOF and RBV was safe and well tolerated. High SVR rates across multiple HCV genotypes were achieved by patients with advanced cirrhosis CTP class A and B or post-liver transplant, but not in CTP class C pre-liver transplant

Expanded Access Programme Cohort Study

Foster GR, Irving WL, Cheung MC, et al. Impact of direct acting antiviral therapy in patients with chronic hepatitis C and decompensated cirrhosis. *J Hepatol.* 2016 Jun;64(6):1224–1231.

Study description: Open-label, observational cohort study of the Expanded Access Programme (EAP)

Patient population: TN patients with HCV and decompensated cirrhosis ($n = 467$, 87% decompensated cirrhosis) versus retrospective comparator cohort ($n = 261$)

Study arms: Treatment cohort was enrolled before treatment through the EAP and followed prospectively for 6 months after treatment completion. Comparator untreated cohort was identified retrospectively in the United Kingdom HCV Research Database. Primary endpoint was SVR12 (treated cohort), and the secondary endpoint (both cohorts) was adverse outcomes (worsening MELD score or serious adverse event) within 6 months of treatment or monitoring. DAAs administered: LED/SOF or SOF/DCV given with or without RBV for 12 weeks

Results/SVR12:

GT1: 90.5%; GT3: 68.8%

Delta-MELD for treated patients was –0.85 (SD 2.54) versus 0.75 (SD 3.54) in untreated cohort

5.6% of patients discontinued therapy with 3.6% mortality rate in treatment group as compared to 5.7% in the untreated cohort

Overall outcome of adverse events and worsening of MELD score: 52.3% in the treated cohort; 63.6% in the untreated cohort

Significance: DAA therapy is highly effective in patients with decompensated HCV cirrhosis, with a small increase in risk of mortality. Furthermore, improvement in liver function was seen within 6 months of viral clearance as compared to untreated patients.

SOLAR-2 Trial

Manns M, Samuel D, Gane EJ, et al. Ledipasvir and sofosbuvir plus ribavirin in patients with genotype 1 or 4 hepatitis C virus infection and advanced liver disease: a multicenter, open-label, randomised, phase 2 trial. *Lancet Infect Dis.* 2016 Jun;16(6):685–697.

Study description: Randomized, multicenter, open-label, prospective study, phase II

Patient population: HCV GT1 ($n = 296$) or GT4 ($n = 37$). No prior exposure to NS5A inhibitor

Study arms: Cohort A = pretransplant CTP Class B or C cirrhosis

Cohort B = posttransplantation patients with or without cirrhosis; CTP-A, CTP-B cirrhosis, or CTP-C fibrosing cholestatic hepatitis. Fixed-dose combination of LED/SOF plus RBV for 12 weeks (Arm 1) or 24 weeks (Arm 2)

Results/SVR12:
Cohort A: GT1
Arm 1, 87% in CTP-B; Arm 2, 96%
Arm 1, 85% in CTP-C; Arm 2, 78%
Cohort B
GT1: 93% in patients without cirrhosis for 12 weeks; 100% for 24 weeks
Arm 1: 100% in CTP-A; Arm 2, 96%
Arm 1: 95% in CTP-B; Arm 2, 100%
Arm 1: 50% in CTP-C; Arm 2, 80%
SVR12 100% in all five patients with fibrosing cholestatic hepatitis
GT4, SVR12 with 12 weeks was 78% and 94% with 24 weeks of treatment
2% discontinuations due to adverse events; 5% deaths due to complications of hepatic decompensation
Significance: Established the efficacy of LED/SOF with RBV in patients with decompensated cirrhosis and advanced liver disease pre- and post-liver transplantation.

Posttransplant

CORAL-1 Trial

Kwo PY, Mantry PS, Coakley E, et al. An interferon-free antiviral regimen for HCV after liver transplantation. *N Engl J Med*. 2014 Dec 18;371(25):2375–2382.

Study description: Open-label, single-arm, phase II.
Patient population: Chronic HCV infection with GT1 ($n = 34$)
Study arms: Liver transplantation due to HCV at least 12 months prior; TN after transplantation; pretransplant treatment with PEG-IFN + RBV allowed. OBV/PTV/r + dasabuvir + RBV given for 24 weeks
Results/SVR12:
SVR12 and SVR24: 97%
Serious adverse events: 6%; discontinuation: 2.9%
Significance: Established the efficacy of the above regimen among liver transplant recipients with recurrent HCV GT1 infection, a historically difficult-to-treat population.

SOLAR-1 Trial

Charlton M, Everson GT, Flamm SL, et al. Ledipasvir and sofosbuvir plus ribavirin for treatment of HCV infection in patients with advanced liver disease. *Gastroenterology*. 2015 Sep;149(3):649–659.

See the section on Decompensated Liver Disease.

ALLY-1 Trial

Poordad F, Schiff ER, Vierling JM, et al. Daclatasvir with sofosbuvir plus ribavirin for hepatitis C virus infection with advanced cirrhosis or post-liver transplantation recurrence. *Hepatology*. 2016 May;63(5):1493–1505.

See section on Decompensated Liver Disease.

SOLAR-2 Trial

Manns M, Samuel D, Gane EJ, et al. Ledipasvir and sofosbuvir plus ribavirin in patients with genotype 1 or 4 hepatitis C virus infection and advanced liver disease: a multicenter, open-label, randomised, phase 2 trial. *Lancet Infect Dis*. 2016 Jun;16(6):685–697.

See Section on Decompensated Liver Disease.

GALAXY Trial

O'Leary JG, Fontana RJ, Brown K, et al. Efficacy and safety of simeprevir and sofosbuvir with and without ribavirin in subjects with recurrent genotype 1 hepatitis C post-orthotopic liver transplant: the randomized GALAXY study. *Transpl Int.* 2017 Feb;30(2):196–208.

Study description: Randomized, prospective, phase II
Patient population: Recurrent HCV GT1 without cirrhosis ($n = 46$)
Study Arm: Randomized 1:1:1 into three arms (stratified by GT/subtype and Q80K): Arm 1: SIM + SOF + RBV, 12 weeks; Arm 2: SIM+ SOF, 12 weeks; Arm 3: SIM + SOF, 24 weeks (included 13 additional patients, 2 with cirrhosis)
Results/SVR12:
Arm 1: 81.8%; Arm 2: 100%; Arm 3: 93.9%
One viral relapse (follow-up week 4; Arm 1)
Significance: SIM/SOF for 12 weeks without RBV was highly effective in post-liver transplant HCV recurrence. Neither extending treatment to 24 weeks nor adding RBV improved SVR in GT1 HCV post-liver transplant patients.

HIV Coinfection

PHOTON-1 Trial

Sulkowski MS, Naggie S, Lalezari J, et al. Sofosbuvir and ribavirin for hepatitis C in patients with HIV coinfection. *JAMA.* 2014 Jul 23–30;312(4):353–361.

Study description: Open-label, observational, phase III
Patient population: GT1 (TN), GT2, GT3 (TN or TE) HCV with HIV coinfection on stable HAART with CD4 >200 or untreated with CD4 >500, up to 20% cirrhosis ($n = 223$)
Study arms: 24 weeks of SOF plus RBV for GT1 or TE GT2 and GT3, 12 weeks for TN GT2 and GT3
Results/SVR12:
TN GT1: 76%; GT2: 88%; GT3: 67%
TE GT2: 92%; GT3: 94%
3% discontinuation due to adverse events.
Significance: The combination of SOF and RBV is effective in patients coinfected with HIV and HCV with an additional benefit in extending treatment to 24 weeks in patients with GT3 HCV infection.

PHOTON-2 Trial

Molina JM, Orkin C, Iser DM, et al. Sofosbuvir and ribavirin for treatment of hepatitis C virus in patients co-infected with HIV (PHOTON-2): a multicentre, open-label, non-randomised, phase 3 study. *Lancet.* 2015 Mar 21; 385(9973):1098–1106.

Study description: Open-label, observational, phase III
Patient population: TN GT1, GT2, GT3, and GT4 and TE GT2, GT3 with HIV (on antiretroviral therapy [ART] with HIV RNA ≤50 copies/mL and CD4 >200 cells/mm^3) coinfection, up to 20% with cirrhosis ($n = 274$)
Study arms: 12 weeks of SOF and weight-based RBV for TN GT2, 24 weeks for all others

Results/SVR12:
GT1: 85%; GT2: 88%; GT3: 89%; GT4: 84%
Similar SVR12 among TN or TE genotypes: >83%
Serious adverse events: 1%; Discontinuation: 2%
Significance: Established that the combination of SOF and RBV can be used to effectively to treat patients with HIV and HCV coinfection. Along with PHOTON 1, confirmed the benefit of extending therapy to 24 weeks for select genotypes or with TE patients.

TURQUOISE-I Trial

Sulkowski MS, Eron JJ, Wyles D, et al. Ombitasvir, paritaprevir co-dosed with ritonavir, dasabuvir, and RBV for hepatitis C in patients co-infected with HIV-1: A randomized trial. *JAMA*. 2015 Mar 24–31;313(12):1223–1231.

Study description: Randomized, open-label, phase II/III
Patient population: TN or TE with HCV GT1 and HIV-1 (CD4$^+$ count of ≥200/mm^3 or ≥14% CD4$^+$ and plasma HIV-1 RNA suppressed while on atazanavir- or raltegravir-inclusive ART) coinfection including those with cirrhosis (19%) ($n = 63$)
Study arms: Randomized as OBV/PTV/r, dasabuvir, and RBV for 12 weeks (Arm 1) or 24 weeks (Arm 2) of treatment
Results/SVR12:
Arm 1: 94%; Arm 2: 91%
Serious adverse events: 3% in each arm with no discontinuations
Significance: Established the efficacy of the above regimen among patients coinfected with HCV GT1 and HIV-1 with cirrhosis without benefit of extending the therapy to 24 weeks.

C-EDGE Coinfection Trial

Rockstroh JK, Nelson M, Katlama C, et al. Efficacy and safety of grazoprevir (MK-5172) and elbasvir (MK-8742) in patients with hepatitis C virus and HIV co-infection: A non-randomised, open-label trial. *Lancet HIV*. 2015 Aug;2(8):e319–327.

Study description: Observational, open-label, single-arm, phase III
Patient population: TN patients with chronic HCV GT1, GT4, or GT6 infection and HIV (stable on any ART for at least 8 weeks) coinfection with ($n = 35$) or without cirrhosis ($n = 183$)
Study arms: All patients received GZR/EBR for 12 weeks
Results/SVR12:
Overall: 96.3%
GT1a: 96.5%; GT1b: 95.5%; GT4: 96.4%
Cirrhosis: 100%; noncirrhosis: 95.6%
No drug-related serious adverse events or discontinuations, although overall 2% patients had virologic relapse while 1% had reinfection
Significance: The study proved the efficacy of the above regimen in cirrhotic and noncirrhotic patients coinfected with HCV and HIV.

ALLY-2 Trial

Wyles DL, Ruane PJ, Sulkowski MS, et al. Daclatasvir plus sofosbuvir for HCV in patients coinfected with HIV-1. *N Engl J Med*. 2015 Aug 20;373(8):714–725.

Study description: Randomized, multicenter, open-label, phase III

Patient population: TE (excluding NS5A inhibitors) (*n* = 151) or TN (*n* = 52) HCV GT1, GT2, GT3, or GT4, HIV (stable ART with HIV RNA <50 copies/mL at screening and <200 copies/mL for ≥8 weeks and CD4 count >100 cells/mm^3), with or without cirrhosis (<50%) (*N* = 395)

Study arms: 2:1 randomization: cirrhotic or noncirrhotic, TN 12 weeks (Arm 1) or 8 (Arm 2) weeks of DCV and SOF daily while TE patients assigned 12 weeks (Arm 3) of therapy

Results/SVR12:

Overall SVR12 across all GTs in three arms were 97.0%, 76.0%, and 98.1%, respectively

GT1: Arm 1: 96.4%; Arm 2: 75.6%; Arm 3: 97.7% (GT1a and 1b: >96% in Arms 1 and 3 while <80% in Arm 2)

GT2, 3, 4: Arms 1 and 3: 100%; Arm 2: <83%

Overall SVR12 in Arms 1 and 3: 92% with cirrhosis; 98% without cirrhosis; Arm 2: overall <78% with or without cirrhosis

No serious adverse events or discontinuations due to study drugs

Significance: Established the efficacy of DCV/SOF for 12 weeks in HCV and HIV-1 coinfected patients.

ION-4 Trial

Naggie S, Cooper, C, Saag M, et al. Ledipasvir and sofosbuvir for HCV in patients coinfected with HIV-1. *NEJM* 2015; 373:705–713.

Study description: Open-label, multicenter, phase III

Patient population: HCV and HIV coinfection, GT1 (98%) and GT4 TN or TE (55%), with or without cirrhosis, CD4 >100 cells/mm^3, HIV RNA <50 copies/mL, HAART tenofovir-emtricitabine plus efavirenz or rilpivirine or raltegravir allowed (*n* = 335)

Study arms: 12-week course of LED/SOF

Results/SVR12:

Overall 96%

TN: 95%; TE: 97%

Cirrhosis: 94%; no cirrhosis: 96%

2% of patients with serious adverse events with no discontinuations

Significance: Established the efficacy of the regimen of LED/SOF for 12 weeks in HCV GT1 or GT4 patients coinfected with HIV-1.

ASTRAL 5 Trial

Wyles D, Brau N, Kottilil S, et al. Sofosbuvir and velpatasvir for the treatment of hepatitis C virus in patients coinfected with human immunodeficiency virus type 1: An open-label, phase III study. *Clin Infect Dis*. 2017 Mar 29.

Study description: Single-arm, open-label, phase III

Patient population: HCV (CD4 count ≥100 cells/mm^3, HIV RNA ≤50 copies/mL; on stable ART for ≥ 8 weeks) and HIV coinfection; GT1, GT2, GT3, GT4, or GT6 TN or TE, except with NS5A or NS5B (29%), with (18%) or without compensated cirrhosis (*n* = 106)

Study arms: SOF/VEL for 12 weeks:

Results/SVR12:

Overall 95%

GT1a: 95%; GT1b: 92%; GT2: 100%; GT3: 92%; GT4: 100%

TN: 93%; TE: 97%
Cirrhosis: 100%; no cirrhosis: 94%
Serious adverse event: 2%; discontinuation: 2%
Significance: Established the pan-genotypic efficacy of the regimen of sofobuvir plus velpatasvir for 12 weeks in HCV-HIV coinfected patients.

Renal Disease
C-SURFER Trial
Roth D, Nelson DR, Bruchfeld A, et al. Grazoprevir plus elbasvir in treatment-naive and treatment-experienced patients with hepatitis C virus genotype 1 infection and stage 4-5 chronic kidney disease (the C-SURFER study): A combination phase 3 study. *Lancet*. 2015 Oct 17;386(10003):1537–1545.

Study description: Randomized, observational, phase III
Patient population: TN (80%) or TE (19%) HCV GT1 infection with chronic kidney disease (CKD) (stage 4–5, 76% on hemodialysis) and cirrhosis (6%) ($N = 235$)
Study arms: Patients randomly assigned to the immediate treatment group (ITG) ($n = 111$) or the deferred treatment group ($n = 113$), and intensive pharmacokinetic population (PK) ($n = 11$). GZR/EBR was administered for 12 weeks. Patients in the deferred treatment group (DTG) received GZR/EBR regimen after 4 weeks of follow-up and unmasking
Results/SVR12:
SVR12 99%: Combined in the ITG and PK groups in the modified full analysis set
GT1a: 100%; GT1b: 98.2%
Cirrhosis: 100%: no cirrhosis: 99.1%
TN: 100%; TE: 95%
On dialysis: 98.9%; no dialysis: 100%
ITG group only: Relapse: 1%
DTG group only: Serious adverse events: 1%; discontinuation: 4.4%
Deaths: ITG group: 0.8%; DTG group: 2.7%
Significance: Established the efficacy of the regimen of GZR plus EBR for 12 weeks in patients infected with HCV GT1 and stage 4–5 CKD with or without dialysis.

RUBY-I Trial
Pockros PJ, Reddy KR, Mantry PS, et al. Efficacy of direct-acting antiviral combination for patients with hepatitis C virus GT1 infection and severe renal impairment or end-stage renal disease. *Gastroenterology*. 2016 Jun;150(7):1590–1598.

Study description: Multicenter, single-arm, phase IIIb
Patient population: TN adults with HCV GT1 infection without cirrhosis and CKD stage 4 (30%) or 5, including those on dialysis (70%) ($N = 20$)
Study arms: Administered OBV/PTV/r with dasabuvir for 12 weeks. Patients with HCV GT1a infections also received RBV ($n = 13$), but not those with GT1b infection ($n = 7$).
Results/SVR12:
SVR12: 90%

Relapse: 5%; deaths: 5%

Significance: Established the efficacy of the regimen of OBV/PTV/r with dasabuvir among patients with HCV GT1 infection and CKD stage 4 or 5.

RUBY-II Trial

Gane E. RUBY-II: Efficacy and safety of a RBV-free ombitasvir/paritaprevir/ritonavir ± dasabuvir regimen in patients with severe renal impairment or end-stage renal disease and HCV genotypes 1a or 4 infection. AASLD Liver*Learning* Nov 12, 2016;143829.

RUBY-II is an open-label, multicenter phase IIIb trial which evaluated the regimen of OBV/PTV/r ± dasabuvir in noncirrhotic TN patients ($n = 18$) with HCV GT1a or GT4 infection with end-stage renal disease (ESRD) on dialysis. Study Arm 1 comprised patients with HCV GT1a who received OBV/PTV/r and DSV for 12 weeks ($n = 13$) while Arm 2 comprised patients with HCV GT4 who received OBV/PTV/r without DSV for 12 weeks ($n = 5$). Overall SVR12 was 94% in ITT population, with 100% SVR12 among the GT1a patients and 80% SVR12 among the GT4 patients. Overall SVR12 was 94% in ITT population, with 100% SVR12 among the GT1a patients and 80% SVR12 among the GT4 patients. No serious adverse events were noted due to the study drugs, although 8% in Arm 1 and 20% in Arm 2 discontinued therapy owing to the adverse events. The preliminary results of this study establish the efficacy of the regimen of OBV/PTV/r ± dasabuvir for 12 weeks in HCV GT1a or GT4 noncirrhotic TN patients with ESRD on dialysis.

EXPEDITION-4 Trial

Gane E, Lawitz E, Pugatch D, et al. Glecaprevir and pibrentasvir in patients with HCV and severe renal impairment. *NEJM*. 2017;377(15):1448–1455.

EXPEDITION-4 is an multicenter, open-label, single-arm, phase III trial which evaluated the efficacy of the regimen GLE/PIB for 12 weeks in TN or TE patients with GT1–GT6 HCV infection with (19%) or without cirrhosis (81%) and ESRD with 82% on dialysis ($n = 104$). 98% SVR12 was observed in ITT with no virologic failures, although 4% of discontinuation was observed due to adverse events. These preliminary results establish GLE/PIB to be effective and well-tolerated among patients with HCV infection and CKD stage 4 or 5 and on dialysis

Prior DAA Failure

GS-US-342-1553 Study

Gane EJ, Shiffman ML, Etzkorn K, et al. Sofosbuvir/velpatasvir in combination with ribavirin for 24 weeks is effective retreatment for patients who failed prior NS5A containing DAA regimens: Results of the GS-US-342-1553 study. *J Hepatol*. 2016;64(2):S147–S148.

Study description: Single-arm, open-label, phase II
Patient population: TE patients with SOF/VEL or SOF/VEL/VOX with HCV GT1, GT2, or GT3, with or without cirrhosis ($n = 41$)
Study arms: SOF/VEL+RBV for 24 weeks

Results/SVR12:

GT3: SVR12 100% in patients without NS5A RAVs; 77% among those with NS5A RAV

6% in HCV GT1 and GT2

Significance: Established the efficacy of SOF/VEL plus RBV for 24 weeks in patients who previously failed prior SOF/VEL containing regimens despite RAVs.

ANRS HC34 REVENGE Trial

De Ledinghen V, Laforest C, Hezode C, et al. Retreatment with sofosbuvir plus grazoprevir/elbasvir plus ribavirin of patients with hepatitis C virus genotype 1 or 4 who previously failed an NS5A or NS3-containing regimen. ANRS HC34 REVENGE. *Clin Infect Dis*. 2017 Oct 25. [Epub ahead of print].

REVENGE is an open-label, randomized trial which studied the hepatitis C patients carrying resistance associated substitutions (RASs). The study evaluated the regimen of SOF + GZR + EBR + RBV for 16 vs. 24 weeks in TE (SOF plus SIM/DCV/LED with or without RBV) cirrhotic HCV GT1 or GT4 patients with NS5A or NS3 RASs ($n = 26$). SVR4 was established as the secondary endpoint to assess the antiviral efficacy. Overall, 92% patients had NS5A RASs and 8% had NS3 RAS. In this preliminary analysis, SVR4 was 94% according to the data availability of only 17 patients as of now. No relapses were observed, although, out of 15% HCC patients, HCC recurrence was seen in 8%. The REVENGE trial established the efficacy of the regimen of SOF + GZR + EBR with RBV for 16 weeks as a promising option in TE cirrhotic patients with NS5A/NS3 RASs.

Magellan-1 Trial

Poordad F, Felizarta F, Asatryan A, et al. Glecaprevir and pibrentasvir for 12 weeks for hepatitis C virus genotype 1 infection and prior direct-acting antiviral treatment. *Hepatology*. 2017 Aug;66(2):389–339.

Study description: Randomized, multicenter, open-label, phase II

Patient population: TE with prior DAA failure (protease inhibitor [PI]-experienced/NS5A-experienced/PI and NS5A-experienced/SOF-experienced), HCV GT1 without cirrhosis. ($n = 50$)

Study arms: Randomization into 1:1:1 stratified by genotype (GT1b or non-1b) and prior treatment. Arm 1: GLE 200 mg + PIB 80 mg; Arm 2: GLE 300 mg + PIB 120 mg + RBV 800 mg; Arm 3: GLE 300 mg + PIB 120 mg)

Results/SVR12:

SVR12 ITT: 100%, 95%, and 86% in the three arms, respectively

Virologic failure: 4% in Arm 2 and 3 among GT1a patients.

Serious adverse events and discontinuation: None related to the study drugs

Significance: Established the efficacy of GLE/PIB for 12 weeks in prior DAA-experienced noncirrhotic GT1 patients despite baseline NS3 and/or NS5A RAVs with no additional benefit on addition of RBV.

Other Interesting Trials

COSMOS Trial

Lawitz E, Sulkowski MS, Ghalib R, et al. Simeprevir plus sofosbuvir, with or without ribavirin, to treat chronic infection with hepatitis C virus genotype 1 in non-responders to pegylated interferon and ribavirin and treatment-naïve patients: The COSMOS randomised study. *Lancet.* 2014 Nov 15;384(9956):1756–1765.

COSMOS is the first trial of a combination all-oral DAA regimen. It is a randomized, open-label, phase IIa trial which studied SIM/SOF with or without RBV in TN or TE HCV GT1 patients with or without cirrhosis ($n = 167$). Cohort 1 included previous nonresponders with METAVIR scores F0–F2, and cohort 2 was composed of previous nonresponders and TN patients with METAVIR scores F3–F4. The patients were randomized into a 2:1:2:1 ratio to SIM/SOF with or without RBV for 12 and 24 weeks. Overall 92% SVR12 was observed in the ITT population, with 90% in cohort 1 and 94% in cohort 2. Also, the presence of Gln80Lys (Q80K) polymorphism did not seem to impact the SVR12. SVR in the 24-week treatment group was not significantly higher even in those with treatment experience or advanced fibrosis. 2% of patients in the 24-week arms receiving SIM/SOF ± RBV developed serious adverse events as compared to none in the 12-week arms. Discontinuation was seen in 2% of patients in all arms. The regimen established its efficacy in TN or TE HCV GT1 patients with F0–F4 fibrosis without significant benefit in extending the therapy to 24 weeks (compare to the OPTIMIST-2 trial in the section "Currently Approved Therapies").

PEARL-I Trial

Hézode C, Asselah T, Reddy KR, et al. Ombitasvir plus paritaprevir plus ritonavir with or without ribavirin in treatment naive and treatment experienced patients with genotype 4 chronic hepatitis C virus infection: a randomised, open-label trial. *Lancet.* 2015;385(9986):2502–2509.

PEARL-1, a randomized, multicenter, open-label, phase IIb trial evaluated the efficacy of the regimen of OBV/PTV/r with or without RBV in TN or TE noncirrhotic HCV GT4 patients ($n = 135$). SVR12 of 100% was observed with RBV in TN and TE patients and 91% without RBV in TN patients. Virologic failures were noted in 3% of the patients in the TN arm and none in the TE arm. This study established the superior efficacy of OBV/PTV/r + RBV for treatment of noncirrhotic HCV GT4 patients irrespective of their previous treatment status

BOSON Trial

Foster GR, Pianko S, Brown A, et al. Efficacy of SOF plus RBV with or without peginterferon-alfa in patients with hepatitis C virus genotype 3 infection and treatment-experienced patients with cirrhosis and hepatitis C virus genotype 2 infection. *Gastroenterology.* 2015 Nov;149(6):1462–1470.

BOSON is the first trial to report the efficacy of SOF in a traditionally difficult to treat population. It was a randomized, open-label, phase III trial which studied the efficacy SOF and RBV with or without PEG-IFNα in TN or TE cirrhotic and noncirrhotic HCV GT3 patients and in TE cirrhotic HCV GT2 patients. The randomization was done 1:1:1 to three arms: Arm 1, SOF and RBV for 16 weeks; Arm 2, SOF and RBV for 24 weeks; Arm 3, SOF, PEG-IFNα, and RBV for 12 weeks ($N = 592$). GT2 patients had a higher SVR12 of 100% in Arm 2, unlike in Arm 1 (87%) and Arm 3 (94%). For GT3, overall SVR12 was 71% in Arm 1, 84% in Arm 2, and 93% in Arm 3. Unlike other arms, Arm 3 had a higher SVR12 rate in TN (SVR12 95%) or TE (SVR12 91%) cirrhotic (SVR12 88%) or noncirrhotic (SVR12 95%) GT3 patients, whereas TN noncirrhotic patients showed a better response than the others. Virologic failure was noted in 1% of GT3 patients in Arm 2, with 1% discontinuation overall. Thus, GT2 patients performed better with SOF+RBV with or without PEG-IFNα for 12 or 24 weeks while GT3 patients showed a better response with SOF+RBV+ PEG-IFNα for all patients for 12 weeks of treatment. The study showed that, on addition of PEG-IFNα, high SVR12 rates are produced in difficult to treat patients with HCV GT2 and GT3 infection.

C-EDGE CO-STAR Trial

Dore GJ, Altice F, Litwin AH, et al. Elbasvir-grazoprevir to treat hepatitis C virus infection in persons receiving opioid agonist therapy: A randomized trial. *Ann Intern Med*. 2016 Nov 1;165(9):625–634.

C-Edge Co-Star is a randomized, placebo-controlled, double-blind, phase III trial which evaluated the efficacy of EBR/GZR regimen for 12 weeks in TN HCV GT1, GT4, and GT6 cirrhotic (20%) or noncirrhotic patients receiving opioid agonist therapy (OAT) for 3 months or more, with more than 80% adherent ($n = 301$). The patients were randomized to 2:1 with the ITG receiving EBR/GZR for 12 weeks and the DTG receiving placebo for 12 weeks, no treatment for 4 weeks, then open-label EBR/GZR for 12 weeks. SVR12 was 91.5% in the ITG arm versus 89.5% in the DTG arm. All the genotypes showed a higher SVR12 rate (>91%) except GT6 (<60%). The presence of cirrhosis did not affect the SVR12 (>91%). 62% in the ITG and 53% in the DTG group had a positive drug screen on Day 1. In the ITG group, 93.8% SVR12 was achieved in patients with a negative drug screen, and 90.4% was observed in patients with a positive drug screen. Fewer than 1% patients discontinued the treatment due to adverse events. The study observed high rates of SVR12 despite ongoing drug use, which further supports the removal of drug use as a barrier to IFN-free HCV treatment for patients receiving OAT.

Index

Page numbers followed by *f*, *t*, and *b* refer to figures, tables, and boxes, respectively.

A

AASLD. See American Association for the Study of Liver Diseases
AASLD-IDSA. See American Association for the Study of Liver Diseases and the Infectious Disease Society of America
Acute cellular rejection, 133*f*
Acute hepatic failure (AHF), 44, 46
Acute hepatitis C virus (HCV), 57–62, 65, 66*f*
 aminotransferases and bilirubin, 61
 antibody testing, 61
 clinical features, 59
 defined, 57
 diagnosis, 59–62, 60*b*
 differentiation between chronic and, 68
 disease progression, 23*f*
 estimated incidence of, 13
 incidence, 17, 57–59
 and jaundice, 21*t*, 59, 61
 outcomes of, 58*f*
 pathological evaluation of, 43–46
 post OLT, 134
 recurrence, 135*f*
 serologic pattern of progression to CHC, 22*f*
 serologic pattern of recovering, 22*f*
 sources of infection, 19–20
 spontaneous clearance, 62
 symptoms of, 20
 treatment, 62
 viral load testing, 61–62
Acute viral hepatitis, 44–46
Agate-I trial, 161
Agents under investigation, 165–69
 Glecaprevir/Pibrentasvir, 168–69
 Sofosbuvir + Velpatasvir + Voxilaprevir, 166–68
 Uprifosbuvir + Grazoprevir + Ruzasvir, 165–66
AHF (acute hepatic failure), 44, 46
AI444040, 97*t*
Alanine aminotransferase (ALT), 36
All-oral DAA regimen, 179
All-oral fixed-dose combinations (FDC), 84
All-oral interferon-free therapy, vii
ALLY-1 trial, 98*t*, 100, 163, 170–72
ALLY-2 Trial, 97*t*, 99, 174–75
ALLY-3 trial, 101, 102*t*–103*t*, 105–6, 162
ALLY-3+ trial, 101, 106, 162–63
α-Fetoprotein (AFP), 71
ALT (alanine aminotransferase), 36
American Association for the Study of Liver Diseases (AASLD), 33, 37, 39, 71, 77, 83, 137
American Association for the Study of Liver Diseases and the Infectious Disease Society of America (AASLD-IDSA), 91, 92, 96, 97*t*–98*t*, 99–101, 102*t*–104*t*
Aminotransferase, 36, 61
ANRS HC34 REVENGE Trial, 178
Antiarrhythmics, 94*t*
Antibody testing, 61
Antibacterials, 94*t*
Anticonvulsants, 94*t*
Anti-D immunoglobulin, 21
Antigen detection, HCV core, 36
Anti-HCV antibodies, 20, 21, 35, 43
Anti-HCV seroprevalence, 7, 9*t*
Antiviral drugs, 1
Antiviral therapy, 36, 79, 80
APASL (Asian Pacific Association for the Study of the Liver), 71*t*
Arthralgia, 67*b*
Arthritis, 67*b*
Asian Pacific Association for the Study of the Liver (APASL), 71*t*
Aspartate aminotransferase (AST), 61
ASTRAL-1 Trials, 86, 96, 97*t*, 164
ASTRAL-2 Trials, 96, 97*t*, 99, 164–65
ASTRAL-3 Trials, 101, 102*t*–103*t*, 105–6, 164–65
ASTRAL-4 Trials, 98*t*, 100, 104*t*, 106, 170
ASTRAL-5 Trials, 175–76

B

B-cell lymphoma, 78–79
Bilirubin, 61
Bleeding, variceal, 69, 69*b*, 70
Boceprevir, 38
BOSUN Trials, 179–80

C

Calcineurin inhibitors, 139, 139*t*
Capsid, 1, 2*f*
Carcinoma, hepatocellular. See Hepatocellular carcinoma
C-CREST Trials 1 and 2 Parts A–C, 165–66
CD20 protein, 77
CD81 protein, 78
CDC. See Centers for Disease Control and Prevention
C-EDGE Coinfection Trial, 174
C-EDGE Co-Star trial, 180

C-EDGE Treatment-Experienced Trial, 163–64
C-EDGE Treatment-Naïve Trial, 163
Centers for Disease Control and Prevention (CDC), 20, 33, 35, 39, 65, 66
Chain termination, 5
CHC. See Chronic hepatitis C
Child-Pugh score, 69
Child-Turcotte-Pugh (CTP) score, 112–13, 137
Chronic ductopenic rejection, 134f
Chronic hepatitis C (CHC), 65–72
 cirrhosis with, 25, 71
 clinical presentation, 67–68
 in COSMOS trial, 178–79
 diagnosis of, 36–37
 differentiation between acute and, 68
 disease progression, 21–23, 23f, 43–44, 66f
 fibrosis in, 25, 48f
 follow-up pathological assessment, 49
 genotype 1, 38
 global prevalence of, 8, 10f
 in individuals with HIV, 120–21
 initial pathological assessment, 46–49, 47f
 and jaundice, 68b
 and liver transplantation, 26
 mortality rates, 26
 prevalence in US, 12–13
 risk factors and screening, 66–67
 risk factors for increased fibrosis, 68b
 scope of the problem, 65, 66
 serologic profile of, 34f
 testing for, 33
Cirrhosis, 68–70
 caused by HCV, 7–8
 from CHC, 22–26, 23f, 43, 46, 59, 65, 66f, 71, 91–93
 compensated, 26, 86, 86b–88b, 97t, 105–6, 137–39
 complications of, 69b
 confirmation of, using Masson's trichrome stain, 141f
 decompensated, 50, 51, 67, 84, 85, 98t, 137–38, 169–73
 explanted liver with, 51f
 indicators of, 36, 37
 monitoring complications after cure, 150, 151
 and OLT, 43, 134, 135
 predictors of, 26
 progression of, 1
 progression of fibrosis to, 24–25, 36, 52
 in testing algorithm for HCV, 39f
Computed tomography (CT), 71
CORAL-1 Trial, 172
Corticosteroids, 77, 78f
COSMOS Trial, 178–79
Cryoglobulins, 76–77
C-SURFER Trial, 176
C-SURGE Trial, 166
CT (computed tomography), 71
CTP score. See Child-Turcotte-Pugh score

D

DAAs. See Direct-acting antiviral agents
Daclatasvir, 84, 95, 113, 113t, 115t, 119t, 121t, 122, 139t, 162–63
DCP (des-γ-carboxy prothrombin), 71
Decompensated cirrhosis, 23f, 50, 51
 post OLT, 172–73
 pre OLT, 138, 169–72
 treatment of HCV with, 98t, 100, 104t, 106–7, 111–14, 117
Dermatologic manifestations, 67b
Des-γ-carboxy prothrombin (DCP), 71
Diabetes mellitus, 67b
Diagnostic testing
 antibody testing, 61
 HCV core antigen detection, 36
 HCV genotyping, 36–39
 hepatitis C virus (HCV), 33–39
 liver biopsy, 37
 noninvasive assessment of liver fibrosis, 37–38
 pharmacogenetics testing, 38
 routine laboratory testing, 36
 screening, 33, 66–67
Direct-acting antiviral agents (DAAs)
 with antiviral regimens, 113t
 and b-cell lymphoma, 79
 with decompensated cirrhosis, 111–13
 efficacy of, 43, 142–43
 following liver transplantation, 118, 138–40
 with HCV recurrence, 134–35
 persistence of RAVs following treatment with, 125t
 and porphyria cutanea tarda, 80
 renal excretion of, 115t
 and SVR rates, 81, 83
 treatment with HIV coinfection, 121t
 virological resistance to, 123–26, 124t
Direct-acting antiviral (DAA) therapies, 151–52
 goal of, 149
 and mixed cryoglobulinemia, 75, 77
 new, 89b, 140
 oral combination, 137, 142
 outcomes of, 92–93
Disease progression, HCV, 23–26
 behavioral factors, 25
 demographic factors, 24–25
 genetic factors, 26
 metabolic factors, 25
 viral factors, 26
DNA polymerases, 2, 3
Drug-drug interactions, 118
 between DAAs and immunosuppressants, 119t, 139–40, 139t
 between sofosbuvir and ART regimen agents, 122
Ductulitis, 53

E

E1 protein, 1
E2 protein, 1

EASL. *See* European
Association for
the Study of
the Liver
EIA testing. *See* Enzyme
immunoassay
testing
Elbasvir, 84, 115*t*, 119*t*,
121*t*, 163–64
Elbasvir/grazoprevir, 84,
139*t*, 140, 180
ELISA (enzyme-linked
immunosorbent
assay), 67, 68
Endosomes, 3
Endothelitis, 53
ENDURANCE Trials,
98*t*, 168
Envelope, 1
Enzyme immunoassay (EIA)
testing, 34, 35,
39, 39*f*
Enzyme-linked
immunosorbent
assay (ELISA),
67, 68
Epclusa, 3
Epidemiology of HCV, 7–13
and genotypes, 8, 12
and mutability of HCV
genome, 7
and risk factors for
recurrence,
131–33, 132*t*
in United States, 12–13
worldwide prevalence,
7–8, 9*t*, 10*f*–11*f*
Essential mixed
cryoglobulinemia,
67*b*
EtOH hepatitis, 51
European Association for
the Study of the
Liver (EASL), 71,
71*t*, 91–92, 96,
97*t*–98*t*, 102*t*–104*t*
EXPEDITION 1 Trials, 97*t*,
98*t*, 99
EXPEDITION 4 Trials, 177
Explanted HCV cirrhotic
liver, 44, 51–52,
51*f*, 52*f*
Extrahepatic manifestations
of CHC, 22, 59,
67*b*, 75–81, 76*b*
B-cell lymphoma, 78–79
mixed cryoglobulinemia
(MC), 75–78, 79
multidisciplinary
approach to
treatment of, 80–81
porphyria cutanea tarda
(PCT), 79–80

F

FHN (fulminant hepatic
necrosis), 44, 46
Fibrosing cholestatic hepatitis
(FCH), 44, 53, 53*f*,
140–43, 141*f*
Fibrosis, 36–38, 44, 48, 93,
134–35, 141*f*
noninvasive assessment
of, in liver, 37–38
noninvasive markers of, 34*t*
progression of, to
cirrhosis, 24–25, 36
regression of, 149–50
stage of, 21, 46
FISSION Trial,
94–95, 155–56
Fulminant hepatic necrosis
(FHN), 44, 46
Fulminant hepatitis C, 20
FUSION trial, 96, 156

G

GALAXY Trial, 173
Garnet trial, 162
Genotype(s), HCV,
2–5, 8, 12
relative prevalence
of each by GBD
region, 11*f*
rs8099917 (T/T),
21, 26, 38
rs12979860 (C/C),
21, 26, 38
Genotype 1 (GT1), 26,
36–38, 83–88
CHC, 178–79
with CKD, 116–17
DAA failures, therapies
for, 87, 88, 124
prevalence of, 8, 13, 83
treatment failure to
PEG-IFN + PI for,
87, 87*b*
treatment for
compensated
cirrhosis, 86
decompensated
cirrhosis, 111–14
noncirrhotic, 85
options, 83–87
Genotype 1a (GT1a), 8,
37, 123–24
Genotype 1b (GT1b), 37, 75
Genotype 2 (GT2), 8, 12,
13, 36, 179–80
DAA treatment
regimens, 95–96,
99–101, 117
treatment experienced,
97*t*–98*t*, 99–100

treatment naïve,
96–99, 97*t*
treatment of, 97*t*–98*t*
Genotype 2b (GT2b), 79
Genotype 3 (GT3), 8, 13,
36, 48, 68, 68*b*,
117–18, 179–80
antiviral regimens, 117
DAA treatment
regimens,
93–96, 99–101
and liver disease, 26, 51
pretreatment testing, 92
treatment experienced,
103*t*–104*t*, 105–6
treatment naïve, 101,
102*t*, 105
Genotype 4 (GT4), 12,
13, 179
with CKD, 116–17
treatment options for, 88
Genotype 5 (GT5), 12, 13,
83, 88, 88*b*, 117
Genotype 6 (GT6), 12, 13,
83, 88, 88*b*, 117
Genotype 7 (GT7), 12
Genotyping, HCV, 34*t*,
36–38, 36–39,
68, 68*b*
Glecaprevir, 84, 95, 115*t*,
119*t*, 121*t*, 168–69
Glecaprevir/pibrentasvir, 84,
97*t*–98*t*, 100, 118
Grazoprevir, 84, 115*t*, 119*t*,
121*t*, 163–66
GS-US-342-1553 Study,
177–78
GT1. *See* Genotype 1
GT2. *See* Genotype 2
GT3. *See* Genotype 3
GT4. *See* Genotype 4
GT5. *See* Genotype 5
GT6. *See* Genotype 6
GT7 (genotype 7), 12

H

"Hard to treat" population,
169–78
HBV. *See* Hepatitis B virus
HCC. *See* Hepatocellular
carcinoma
HCV. *See* Hepatitis C virus
HCV RNA negative, 92
HCV RNA positive, 7, 19
HCV test, 153
Hematologic
manifestations, 67*b*
Hemophilia, 18*f*, 20
Hepatic decompensation,
23, 51, 122–23, 135,
137, 149
Hepatic fibrosis, 138–39

Hepatic lobule
  showing focal necrosis, 45f
  showing isolated hepatocyte undergoing apoptosis, 45f
Hepatitis B virus (HBV), 1
  coinfection with HCV, 25, 49–50
  coinfection with HIV, 120
  reactivation, 151–52
Hepatitis C Check, 35
Hepatitis C virus (HCV), 21t
  and accelerated disease progression factors, 23b
  acute (See Acute hepatitis C virus)
  and advanced liver disease, 23
  and AIH, 50
  antibodies, 33–36
    serum, 12
    testing, 61
  antibody-positive, 19
  basic virology, 1–5
  chronic (See Chronic hepatitis C)
  and chronic liver diseases, 25, 44, 50–51
  coinfections, 25, 49–53
  coinfection with HIV, 68, 68b, 120–23, 131, 132, 173–76
  diagnostic testing, 33–36, 34t
  disease progression, 23–26
    behavioral factors, 25
    demographic factors, 24–25
    genetic factors, 26
    metabolic factors, 25
    viral factors, 26
  estimated prevalence of chronic infection, 9t
  and EtOH hepatitis, 51
  fibrosing cholestatic, 140–43
  genome, 2, 3f
  global burden of disease regions, 9t
  and HBV, 25, 49–50
  higher risk groups for reinfection, 152–53
  and HIV, 25, 50
  host response to, 20–23
  and jaundice, 21
  life cycle, 3, 4f
  and liver diseases, 65
  in liver transplantation, 131–43
  maternal-fetal transmission, 19
  and mucosa-associated lymphoid tissue (MALT) lymphoma, 79
  and NAFLD, 51
  natural history, 17–27, 23f
  nosocomial transmission, 19–20
  pretreatment testing, 92
  prevalence by selected groups, 18f
  quasispecies and genotypes, 2–5
  recurrent, 52–53, 136f
  replication, and drug targets, 3–5
  RNA, 12, 20, 21, 21t, 43, 123
    levels, 25, 52
    testing for, 35–36, 39f, 62
  sexual transmission, 18, 19, 60b
  spontaneous clearance, 21–23
  testing algorithm, 39f
  testing and serologies, 20–22, 22f
  transmission risk factors, 17–20
  transmitted by, 7
  treatment for genotypes 2 and 3, 91–107
  vertical transmission, 19
  viremic rate, 9t
  virion, 1, 2f
Hepatocellular carcinoma (HCC), 23f, 26, 51, 65, 69b, 70–72, 91, 137
  in cirrhotic population, 151
  screening and surveillance of, 37, 70–72, 71t
  varices and variceal bleeding, 69–70, 69b
Hepatocellular cholestasis, 44
Herbal supplements, 94t
Highly active antiretroviral therapy (HAART), 25
High-risk populations, 12, 13b
HIV protease inhibitors, 94t
HLA-DQB1, 21
Home Access Health Corp., 35

Human immunodeficiency virus (HIV), 1

I

IDSA (Infectious Diseases Society of America), 83, 137
IDUs (injection drug users), 58–61, 60b
IFN-based regimens, 121
IL-6, 21
IL28b gene, 21, 34t, 38
IL28b polymorphisms, 26
Immune system, 3
Immunosuppressants, use of, in liver transplantation, 119t
Infectious Diseases Society of America (IDSA), 83, 137
Injection drug users (IDUs), 58–61, 60b
Interface hepatitis, 46, 47f
Interferon (IFN)-based HCV therapies, 134–35
Intravenous drug use (IVDU), 17–18, 25
Investigation, agents under, 165–69
  Glecaprevir/Pibrentasvir, 168–69
  Sofosbuvir + Velpatasvir + Voxilaprevir, 166–68
  Uprifosbuvir + Grazoprevir + Ruzasvir, 165–66
ION-2 Trial, 157
ION-3 Trial, 158
ION-4 Trial, 175
ION trials, 157–58
IVDU (intravenous drug use), 17–18, 25

J

Jaundice
  and acute hepatitis C virus (HCV), 59, 61
  and hepatitis C virus (HCV), 21

L

Ledipasvir, 84, 113–14, 113t, 115t, 119t, 121t, 139t, 157–58
Leukocytoclastic vasculitis, 67b
LFT (liver function test), 44, 133
Lichen planus, 67b

Liver biopsy, 37, 38, 44
Liver diseases, concomitant, 151–52
Liver fibrosis, 24f, 37–38
Liver function test (LFT), 44, 133
Liver transplantation
   for CHC, survival rates, 26
   drug-drug interactions, 119t
   Hepatitis C in, 131–43
Lymphoma, 67b

M

MAGELLAN-1 Trial, 178
MAGELLAN-2 Trial, 168–69
Magnetic resonance imaging (MRI), 71
Management of hepatitis C after cure, 149–53
   achieving SVR, 149–50, 150t
   concomitant liver diseases, 151–52
   monitoring cirrhotic complications, 150, 151
MC (mixed cryoglobulinemia), 75–79
MELD. See Model for end-stage liver disease
Membranoproliferative glomerulonephritis, 67b
Membranoproliferative nephritis, 77
Minus strand, 4
Mixed cryoglobulinemia (MC), 75–79
Model for end-stage liver disease (MELD), 112, 123, 137–38
Monoclonal gammopathy, 67b
MRI (magnetic resonance imaging), 71
Myalgia, 67b

N

NAT (nucleic acid testing), 35–36, 43
National Comprehensive Cancer Network (NCCN), 71t
National Health and Nutrition Examination Survey (NHANES), 12, 68
Neuropathy, 67b
Neutrino trial, 155

NHANES (National Health and Nutrition Examination Survey), 12, 68
NHL (non-Hodgkin's lymphoma) patients, 79
NNPIs (non-nucleoside PIs), 84
Non-A, Non-B hepatitis, 1
Non-Hodgkin's lymphoma (NHL) patients, 79
Non-nucleoside PIs (NNPIs), 84
Nonselective β-blockers, 111–12
NPIs (nucleotide PIs), 84
NS3/4A protease inhibitors, 84, 116–17, 124, 124t, 158–69
NS3 protease, 4
NS3 protein, 1, 4
NS4A protein, 4
NS4B protein, 4
NS5A inhibitors, 3–5, 93–95, 94t, 113–14, 124, 124t, 157–69
NS5A protein, 1
NS5A RAVs, 123
NS5A resistance-associated variants (RAVs), 116–17
NS5B inhibitors, 3, 5, 155–62, 164–68
NS5B non-nucleoside polymerase inhibitors, 124t
NS5B nucleotide polymerase inhibitors, 113, 124t
NS5B polymerase inhibitors, 5
NS5B protein, 1, 4, 37
Nucleic acid testing (NAT), 35–36, 43
Nucleoside analogues, 5
Nucleotide analogues, 5
Nucleotide PIs (NPIs), 84

O

OBV/PTV/r, 179
OLT. See Orthotopic liver transplantation
Ombitasvir, 84, 179
Optimist-1 trial, 158
Optimist-2 trial, 159
Orthotopic liver transplantation (OLT), 131–43
   complications and challenges after, 142–43

   diagnosing HCV after, 131–35
   treating HCV, 135–40
      perioperative, 138
      posttransplant, 138–40, 141f
      pretransplant, 136–38
      retransplantation, 140

P

Pan-genotypic anti-viral regimen, 116–17, 140
Pan-genotypic drug classes, 85t
pangenotypic medications, 118
Paritaprevir, 84, 116–17, 179
Pathology of viral hepatitis C, 43–53
   acute, 43–46
   coinfections, 49–53
   follow-up assessment for CHC, 49
   initial assessment for CHC, 46–48, 49t
PCR (polymerase chain reaction), 68
PCT (porphyria cutanea tarda), 67b, 79–80
PEARL-I Trials, 179
PEARL-II Trials, 161
PEARL-III Trials, 160
PEARL-IV Trials, 160
Pegylated-interferon (PEG-IFN), 37, 38, 91–93
Pegylated interferon-α (PEG-IFNα), 83–84
Pharmacogenetics testing, 38
PHOTON-1 Trials, 173
PHOTON-2 Trials, 173–74
Pibrentasvir, 84, 95, 113, 115t, 119t, 121t, 168–69
Piecemeal necrosis, 46, 47f
PIs (protease inhibitors), 37, 137–38
PIVKA II (prothrombin induced by vitamin K absence II), 71
POLARIS-1 Trials, 166–67
POLARIS-2 Trials, 167
POLARIS-3 Trials, 167
POLARIS-4 Trials, 98t, 167–68
Polymerase chain reaction (PCR), 68
Porphyria cutanea tarda (PCT), 67b, 79–80
POSITRON trial, 94–95, 100, 156

Potential drug-drug
	interactions (DDIs),
	84
Prior DAA failure, 177–78
PrOD, 115t, 116–17, 119t,
	121t, 139t, 140
Progression, disease, 23–26
	behavioral factors, 25
	coinfections, 25
	demographic factors,
		24–25
	from fibrosis to cirrhosis,
		24
	genetic factors, 26
	metabolic factors, 25
	viral factors, 26
Protease inhibitors (PIs),
	37, 137–38
Proteases, 4
Prothrombin induced by
	vitamin K absence II
	(PIVKA II), 71

Q

Quasispecies, HCV, 2–5

R

Radioembolization, 72
Radiofrequency ablation
	(RFA), 72
RAVs, 123–26
Raynaud's phenomenon,
	67b
REALIZE trial, 38
Receptors, 3
Recombinant immunoblot
	assay (RIBA-2 or
	RIBA-3), 35
Recurrent HCV
	in liver transplant
		recipients, 117–20
	in OLT graft, 44, 52–53
Renal disease, 93, 107,
	114, 176–77
Renal manifestations, 67b
Retreatment of HCV, after
	failed previous
	antiviral regimens,
	123–26
Rheumatologic
	manifestations, 67b
Ribavirin (RBV), 37, 38,
	77, 83–84, 92–93,
	95–96, 113, 113t,
	115–17, 137,
	178–80, 179
Ribonucleic acid (RNA),
	1–5. See also specific
	headings, e.g.:
	HCV RNA

Ritonavir, 84, 122, 179
Rituximab, 77, 79
RUBY-I Trial, 176–77
RUBY-II Trial, 177
Ruzasvir, 165–66

S

Sapphire-I trial, 159
Sapphire-II trial, 159–60
Scoring system for grading
	and staging, 49t
Screening, diagnostic,
	33, 66–67
Serial endoscopic variceal
	ligation (EVL), 70
Seronegative window, 62
Sexual transmission
	risk factors, 18,
	19, 60b
Sicca syndrome, 67b
Side effects, adverse
	of corticosteroids, 77
	of daclatasvir, 95
	of PEG-IFN + RBV
		therapy, 92–93,
		95–96, 100–101
	of PEG-IFNα + RBV
		therapy, 83–84
	of ribavirin, 93, 96
	of sofusbuvir, 93
Simprevir, 84, 115t,
	116–17, 119t,
	121t, 138, 139t,
	158–59, 178–79
Single nucleotide
	polymorphisms
	(SNPs), 21
Sofosbuvir (SOF), 137
	and DCV, 142
	drug-drug interactions
		with, 94t, 122, 139t
	and LDV, 142
	trials, 155–59,
		164–68, 178–79
	used with daclatasvir, 84,
		96, 97t–98t, 100,
		113t, 137
	used with ledipasvir, 84,
		113t, 137
	used with RBV, 95–96
	used with simprevir, 84,
		142, 178–79
	used with velpatasvir,
		84, 94–96, 97t–98t,
		100, 113t, 137, 140
	used with velpatasvir and
		voxilaprevir, 84
Sofosbuvir (Sovaldi), 84,
	93–95, 94t, 113–18,
	113t, 115t, 119t,
	121t, 178–80

Sofosbuvir-velpatasvir (SOF
	+ VEL), 84, 94–95,
	113t, 137, 140
SOLAR-1 Trial, 169–70, 172
SOLAR-2 Trial,
	170–71, 172
Spontaneous clearance
	of acute hepatitis C
		virus, 62
	of HCV, 21–23
"Spotty hepatitis," 44,
	45f, 46, 52
SURVEYOR-2 trials, 97t, 99
Sustained virologic
	response (SVR)
	achieved with DAA
		regimens, 86, 87
	achieved with DAAs,
		43–44
	with b-cell lymphoma, 78
	benefits of, 111, 149–50
	and DAAs, 81, 113–14,
		135–40, 142–43
	and genotypes, 91
	and GT1, 83–89
	and GT1a patients,
		125–26, 167, 177
	and GT1 patients, 116,
		166, 179
	for GT2 and GT3
		patients, 92–93, 166
	for GT2 patients, 95–96,
		97t–98t, 99–100
	for GT3 patients, 100–101,
		102t–104t, 105–7
	and GT4 patients,
		177, 179
	and HCC, 151
	for HCV and HIV
		coinfection,
		121–22, 121t
	and IFN-based regimens,
		112
	and liver transplantation,
		118, 170
	with mixed
		cryoglobulinemia,
		75, 77
	monitoring patients after
		achieving, 150,
		150t, 152–53
	with porphyria cutanea
		tarda, 80
	rate of resolution after
		cure, 49
	rates with PEG-IFN,
		38, 84
	and RAVs, 164
	recurrent HCV with
		clinical, 53
	reduced risk of
		developing HCC, 70

T

TECHNIVIE, 159–62
Telaprevir, 38
Therapies, currently approved, 155–65
  Declatasvir, 162–63
  Simeprevir + Sorosbuvir, 158–59
  Sofosbuvir, 155–57
  Sofosbuvir + Ledipasvir, 157–58
  Sofosbuvir + Velpatasvir, 164–65
  Viekira Pak, 159–62
  Zepatier, 163–64
Thrombocytopenia, 36
Transarterial chemo-embolization (TACE), 72
Transmission risk factors
  chronic hepatitis C, 66–67
  injection drug use, 60b
  IV drug use, 17
  nosocomial, 19–20
  sexual, 18, 19, 60b
  unhygenic cosmetic procedures, 17
  vertical (maternal-fetal), 19
Treatment, HCV
  acute HCV, 62
  with advanced CKD, 114–17
  with decompensated cirrhosis, 111–14, 117
  genotype 3 in special populations, 111–26
  genotypes 1, 4, 5, 6, 83–89
  genotypes 2 and 3, 91–107
  with OLT, 135–40
Tumor markers, 71
  Des-γ-carboxy prothrombin (DCP), 71
  α-fetoprotein (AFP), 71
TURQUOISE-I trial, 174
TURQUOISE-II trial, 160
TURQUOISE-III trial, 161

U

Uprifosbuvir, 165–66
US Centers for Disease Control (CDC), 18, 57
US Food and Drug Administration (FDA), 3, 35, 151
US Preventative Services Task Force (USPSTF), 66–67
Uveitis, 67b

V

Valence trials, 96, 100–101, 156–57
Variceal bleeding, 69, 69b, 70
Varices, 69, 70
Velpatasvir, 84, 113, 113t, 115t, 121t, 139t, 164–68
VIEKIRA PAK, 159–62
Viral load testing, 61–62
Virology, HCV, 1–5
Vitamin K, 71
Voxilaprevir, 84, 115t, 166–68

W

World Health Organization (WHO), 65

Z

Zepatier, 163–64

www.ingramcontent.com/pod-product-compliance
Ingram Content Group UK Ltd.
Pitfield, Milton Keynes, MK11 3LW, UK
UKHW061223180426
11947UKWH00027B/1983